"I feel that this book is very up to date...written with a great deal of sensitivity and yet is very clear....It provides important practical information concerning sexuality that every woman ought to be aware of....It is well balanced so that the believer in hormones and the nonbeliever in hormone-replacement therapy can feel equally at home with the subject...."
—ISAAC SCHIFF, M.D., CHIEF OF VINCENT MEMORIAL GYNECOLOGY SERVICE, THE WOMEN'S CARE DIVISION OF THE MASSACHUSETTS GENERAL HOSPITAL, HARVARD MEDICAL SCHOOL

"Menopause is...a natural transitional process that affects body, mind, and soul. To manage this transition well, we need the courage to take responsibility for making our own personal health decisions....Dr. Wulf H. Utian and Ruth S. Jacobowitz have crafted a book that opens our minds to much that is happening in this field....They have achieved remarkable balance where many others have relied on irresponsible rhetoric. *Managing Your Menopause* is well worth exploring for both men and women who are interested in changing their own attitude about this human reality."
—DAGMAR I. CELESTE, FIRST LADY, STATE OF OHIO

"...a much-needed aid to women who are confused about menopause....explains in a clear and understanding manner material which women want to get directly. Estrogen is handled beautifully, giving women the facts but allowing them to decide for themselves....I will be recommending this book to my patients."
—PENELOPE RUSSIANOFF, PH.D., AUTHOR OF *WHEN AM I GOING TO BE HAPPY?* AND *WHY DO I THINK I AM NOTHING WITHOUT A MAN?*

"There is so much valuable information and advice packed into these pages that you will want to refer to it again and again."
—BARBARA L. DRINKWATER, PH.D., DEPARTMENT OF MEDICINE, PACIFIC MEDICINE CENTER, SEATTLE

MANAGING YOUR
Menopause

Wulf H. Utian, M.D., Ph.D., and Ruth S. Jacobowitz

A FIRESIDE BOOK
Published by Simon & Schuster
New York London Toronto Sydney Tokyo Singapore

The case studies included in this book have been altered to protect
the identity of the individuals concerned. Fictitious names have
been used, and composite accounts have been created from the
author's clinical experience.

The ideas, procedures, and suggestions contained in this book are
not intended to replace the services of a trained health professional.
All matters regarding your health require medical supervision. You
should consult your physician before adopting the procedures in this
book. Any applications of the treatments set forth in this book are at
the reader's discretion.

FIRESIDE
Simon & Schuster Building
Rockefeller Center
1230 Avenue of the Americas
New York, New York 10020

FIRESIDE and colophon are registered
trademarks of Simon & Schuster Inc.

Manufactured in the United States of America

10   9   8   7

First Fireside Edition 1992

Library of Congress Cataloging-in-Publication Data
Utian, Wulf H., 1939–
Managing your menopause/Wulf H. Utian and Ruth S.
Jacobowitz.—1st Prentice Hall Press ed.
p.   cm.
1. Menopause—Popular works.   2. Middle-aged women—Health
and hygiene.   I. Jacobowitz, Ruth S.   II. Title.
RG186..U86   1990   80 261111
618.1'75—dc20   CIP

ISBN: 0-671-76426-8

*This book is dedicated
to our spouses, to our children,
and to the good health
of women everywhere.*

Acknowledgments

The preparation of a book such as this one requires the unique contributions of many other persons. Few, if any authors, work in a vacuum or exist in a time warp while their project is underway. For us it was always necessary to carve out extra time for "the book." With sincere appreciation, we want to thank the following important people in our lives.

Wulf Utian thanks "Moira for enormous sacrifices as I work at multiple projects; Brett and Lara for the time I missed with them and Lara for creating and checking the glossary; my scientific colleagues worldwide for shared ideas; my patients for being open, honest, and often instructive."

Ruth Jacobowitz thanks "Paul for his limitless support, time, and understanding and for always believing in me; Lowell for all his patience as he made me computer literate; Julie for her help and time; Alvin, Jan, Jeffrey, Jody, David, Claire Michelle, my mother and sisters, Harriet and Susan, and the Jacobowitz family for being gracious when family time was used for project time; and Marrie for her guidance."

We both would like to thank our editor Toni Sciarra for her timely and thoughtful assistance and Dan MaGurick, our medical illustrator, and Nancy Murray of Fifi Oscard Associates, our agent, who turned our visions into reality.

writer and vice-president for public affairs of a prestigious hospital, surrounded by doctors—without a clue about what was happening to me.

In 1982, three years before that night of panic, I began to plan my early, early retirement. By the summer of 1984, when I gave six months notice, I felt shaky most of the time. Nonetheless, when I left the hospital after eighteen years, it was with a consulting contract in my pocket. Many of the physicians had also asked me to handle their public relations programs. I felt odd, but life still looked good. My husband and I enjoyed a long beach vacation, coming home for the birth of our grandson.

My life came apart one week later. On that terrifying night in 1985, no longer able to contain the panic and sleeplessness, I called a doctor—one who did not move in our social circle. After a physical with blood tests that indicated that I was only "borderline" menopausal, I was treated with an array of tranquilizers, antidepressants, antianxiety drugs, and psychotherapy. But I wasn't getting better. The sleeplessness continued, and all those waking hours could not be filled with television or books. The colors on the TV seemed to run together and I could not concentrate. Reading was an incomprehensible task. Music sounded discordant and made me even more nervous. I could not eat.

I had plenty of consulting work to do, and although I tried hard to be productive, my days were as impossible as my nights. It literally took me hours to decide what to wear and hours more to dress. It took me a full day to write a single paragraph. My husband and my family tried hard to understand and to help. Friends made me try to take bridge lessons, work out, and jog. They all supported me, but all were floundering in confusion, as I was.

One day, while working at the hospital, I was trying to appear "normal" and researching an article that took me to Dr. Wulf Utian's offices. Dr. Utian was known to all as one of the foremost menopause experts in the world. He and I had worked together for years and I had written often of his expertise, but had never related it to me, probably because "I was too young for menopausal problems." As soon as I described to him what was happening to me, however, Dr. Utian ordered a blood test. It was then that I finally learned that I lacked sufficient estrogen. Dr. Utian, my coworker and friend, took over. He prescribed estrogen orally and, briefly, vaginally as well. And he reassured me that I was not "crazy." I had not had a "breakdown." After a couple of weeks of hormone replacement therapy, I

A Very Personal Note

It is March 3, 1985. I am fifty-one years old. I go to bed happily discussing things with my husband: our newly arrived first grandchild, an overseas trip, the time that we finally have for ourselves. At 3:00 A.M., I awake panic-stricken, with my heart pounding. I am afraid to go back to sleep. I feel terror and a detached hostility, which I continue to feel, to a greater or lesser degree, for the next six weeks. I feel, literally, *nothing* else: no warmth or cold, no joy or sadness. I cannot even cry.

I did not think of menopause at all, let alone consider it as the cause. My uterus had been removed when I was in my early forties, so my periods were a thing of the past. With my uterus gone, I lost the usual warning signal of menopause: the cessation of my periods. Since my ovaries were intact, my checkups did not include tests that would have revealed that my hormone levels were dropping. But there were other signals. Several years earlier, I had experienced heart palpitations. When they began on the tennis court, my internist sent me to the hospital for a stress test to look for heart disease. There was none.

I also recalled that many years earlier I began breaking out in a sweat on my face, neck, and scalp on stressful occasions. Often embarrassed by this professionally, I learned simply to wipe my face and go on with whatever I was doing. My silk and nylon nightgowns suddenly made me uncomfortably hot at night. I did not relate this feeling to hot flashes. I did not even bother to describe these strange happenings during my annual gynecological checkups. There were also times when I had a vague suspicion that I could not think quite as clearly or as quickly as I usually did. I attributed it to professional burnout. I never sought a physical reason. Imagine me—for years a medical knew that I was on my way back to a normal life. (For a long time I kept the vast array of tranquilizers and antidepressants that I did not take.)

I remember vividly how it ended. I was jogging in Florida with my daughter on April 19, 1985, just six weeks after the horror had begun. Suddenly, without warning, I felt the warmth of the sun. I felt the touch of the breeze. I felt joy at seeing the boats bobbing in the harbor. *I felt things.* I had become me again.

It took many more months for my fear to dissipate. For the next year, I waited for the other shoe to drop, to discover that this was not a menopausal phenomenon. It never happened, thanks to Dr. Utian's diagnostic genius. No doubt about it—I was better. I remain in good health and happy today, but friends continue to share stories of similar things happening to other friends.

Through my own experience, I became a Utian Menopause Management Program devotee. I still am one. I think quickly and clearly and I keep thinking about other unknowing women and what might be happening to them. Dr. Utian has long been committed to delivering this important information to women everywhere, to let them know that there is a positive way to plan for and enjoy the second half of their lives.

For us, writing this book represents the coming together of the woman medical writer with the devastating menopause experience and the medical expert who has become world-renowned for his pioneering work in improving midlife care for women.

What happened to me should not happen to any woman, anywhere.

—Ruth Jacobowitz
September 1989

Contents

·1·

Living Longer, Living Better

Outwitting the Powerful Ovary

Nancy Norris and Susan Leaf had not seen each other for more than thirty-five years—not since they had tearfully kissed each other good-bye as their parents loaded their Chrysler Town and Country station wagons with the accumulation of four years of memories and memen-tos: the stuff of college life. It was 1954, and Nancy and Susan had graduated from a Big Ten midwestern university after four carefree years. Each left with her bachelor's degree in education, her place on the dean's list, and an engagement ring on the fourth finger of her left hand signifying that she would also get her "Mrs. degree" just as soon as the conflict in Korea ended.

Nancy and Susan had been such close friends from the day they met early in their freshman year that their sorority sisters had nicknamed them "the twins." Both women were blond, blue-eyed, well-built, and slightly more than five feet, five inches tall. They had ample breasts, tiny waists, and doubled their wardrobes by exchanging clothing all the time. They both were outgoing with perky personalities that al-ways attracted a wide entourage of friends.

After graduation, they had returned to their home towns and gotten busy with their own lives. In the first year following graduation, they had telephoned each other frequently. Later, they called only occa-sionally and began to write letters. Letters diminished to infrequent notes and finally to holiday greeting cards, which, when ultimately returned to sender, address unknown, disintegrated into no contact at all.

When the thirty-fifth reunion of the class of 1954 was announced, however, Susan obtained Nancy's current address from her alumni association. They began to write to each other once again in anticipation of their personal reunion. They described their lives, their husband's successes, their children's achievements and problems, and the many activities that had engaged them over the years. They made reservations to share their old room at the sorority house for the reunion weekend. They also made plans for just the two of them to meet first in the coffee shop of the landmark hotel located at the border of the campus.

Imagine Susan's shock and pain when she had difficulty recognizing Nancy among the coffee shop crowd, and for Nancy when she saw her former best friend looking almost exactly as she had remembered her. It was as if the years had stood still for Susan. She had a trim figure, a light step, and a sparkle in her eye. Not so for Nancy. The differences between the "twins" as they recognized each other and hugged were stunning. They knew it.

During the weekend, their sorority sisters could not help noticing the incredible difference between their favorite "twins." Although the aging process had left its mark on all the women to some extent, the changes were most noticeable between Nancy and Susan, perhaps because they had looked so much alike and had been inseparable during their college years.

In fact, the thirty-five intervening years had not dealt with the women fairly. For reasons not obvious to most of the women at the reunion, Nancy now looked approximately twenty years older than Susan. She was three inches shorter in height and was slightly stooped; she was much heavier in weight; her skin was very wrinkled. Behind closed doors and in small groups, their former classmates pondered the subject.

Had Nancy aged more rapidly for genetic reasons? Or, had she been ill? Had Susan been enjoying the benefits of health spas; had she the time to pamper herself constantly; did she have a personal trainer before they had even become vogue? The real reasons for Susan's youthful appearance were apparent only to a few women of the graduating class of 1954. These were the women who had kept fully informed about the scientific advances that were benefiting many women during the female climacteric, or change of life, and menopause. These women knew the reason for the difference between Susan and Nancy: They represented the extremes of ovarian function and ovarian failure.

The Story of Nancy

Nancy Norris was born in North Dakota in 1932 into a loving middle-class family. Her engineer father and her schoolteacher mother had a very difficult time conceiving; therefore, Nancy was an only child. She had a happy childhood and grew up always treated as an equal member of her family. When she left home for college in 1950, it was with the challenge of obtaining her degree in an "appropriate" field for women: teaching, social work, nursing, maybe even journalism; finding the right man to be her future husband, and then beginning her own family unit.

However, fate had decided an unfortunate medical history for Nancy that neither she, her parents, nor her medical practitioners of the time could have foreseen. She was somehow physiologically slated to suffer problems for which medical advancement would arrive too late to help her.

Nancy entered puberty around the usual age of thirteen and experienced her first menstrual period about eighteen months later. At the age of fifteen, her periods, while perfectly regular, became very painful on the first day of menstruation. The pain became so severe that she was taken to see the family physician, who advised her that this experience was normal and prescribed a mild pain-relieving medication. Nancy soon became accustomed to suffering pain one day each month and planned her busy schedule around it. Although this problem sometimes interfered with her activities, she learned to accept and cope with her "bad day."

When she graduated from college, Nancy returned to her home town to teach and to await her fiancé's return from Korea. Two years later, at the age of twenty-four, Nancy experienced a new type of abdominal pain. Previously, the pain had occurred only on the first day of her period. Now she began to feel a nagging pain deep in her lower abdomen and pelvis that began toward the end of her menstrual flow and lasted for several days thereafter.

She went back to her physician and was counseled that the pain was due to the stresses of work coupled with the stress of planning her wedding. The pain persisted. Once again, Nancy learned to cope with it using pain-relieving drugs, although she now often missed a day or two of work each month.

In 1957, at the age of twenty-five, Nancy married her fiancé, Elliot.

They decided that they would like to start raising their family while they were still young, but to their chagrin, Nancy did not become pregnant. The combination of recurring pelvic pain during and following her periods and the problem of infertility eventually convinced Nancy that she should seek specialized medical help. She went to a neighboring town to see a gynecologist.

It was 1958, and gynecological diagnosis and infertility therapy were not very far advanced. Following a full clinical evaluation and an x-ray of her fallopian tubes, the gynecologist advised Nancy that she probably had a medical condition called *endometriosis,* a disease in which tissue that originates as part of the uterine lining becomes embedded in other parts of the pelvis where it does not belong. Because of this condition it would take her unusually long to get pregnant, but the gynecologist said that pregnancy would eventually occur. He told Nancy that surgery to remove the wayward diseased tissue was sometimes attempted, but that he did not recommend it for her.

The following year, a new problem developed. Nancy began to suffer severe pain during intercourse. She began to question her own emotional balance when the gynecologist suggested that her inability to conceive was causing psychosomatic pelvic pain. The pain grew worse and began to cause problems in her marriage. It was not until 1961, when Nancy was twenty-nine and the pain became even more severe, that she was sure the pain was in her body, not in her mind.

Finally, she sought another medical opinion. Her new gynecologist diagnosed the presence of an ovarian cyst and recommended surgery. It was performed immediately and confirmed the diagnosis of endometriosis with large endometriotic cysts that were created from the misplaced tissue located on her right ovary. Her doctor was able to salvage a portion of the right ovary during the conservative surgical procedure. Some of her pain was relieved, but the menstrual agony continued. Nancy still did not conceive, and in 1962 she and Elliot adopted a baby girl.

When she was thirty-four, and had endured ten years of persistent monthly pain, painful intercourse, and an inability to conceive, Nancy had a total hysterectomy that included the removal of both of her ovaries. This surgery relieved the pain, but a new problem developed immediately. Within days of the surgical procedure, Nancy suffered hot flashes. Again, medical advancement and timing were not in her favor. In 1966, physicians worldwide were divided over the question of whether or not to provide postmenopausal estrogen therapy, based on the argument that it interfered with the natural process of aging. Nancy's physician advised her against estrogen therapy, and she was given several medications to help alleviate her symptoms. In the next few years the uncomfortable and embarrassing hot flashes disappeared, but a new problem began to develop. Nancy's vaginal lining was thinning, causing her to experience painful intercourse once again, this time for a different reason.

Nancy and Elliot stayed together because of their daughter, but their sex life ended in 1970 when Nancy was just thirty-eight years old. Unbeknownst to her, Nancy was in an estrogen-deprived state. Along with the thinning of her vaginal lining that had caused the painful intercourse, she was losing tissue from her bone, causing osteoporosis.

When Nancy and Susan met at their thirty-fifth reunion, Nancy had already experienced nineteen years of estrogen deprivation. She had lost a lot of bone and the gradual crushing of her vertebrae had lessened her height by almost three inches. Her skin had thinned and wrinkled. The reason she appeared so aged next to her friend Susan was because of her unfortunate medical problems and medical management and because she crash-dieted often, disdained exercise as an "unladylike" activity, and smoked cigarettes.

No woman today need suffer as Nancy did. Knowledge and help are available to women at midlife.

The Story of Susan

Susan, in contrast, had not only been very lucky but had also taken an active role in determining her own fate. When Susan left college, she moved back home to Cleveland, Ohio, where she taught English in the public school system. She married her fiancé, Jeffrey, and had three children while keeping professionally active. Her love of literature initiated her involvement in the very popular Adult Learning Programs, where groups of men and women met to discuss assigned reading materials. Hers was a morning group made up entirely of women.

Susan became the facilitator in the group. It was within that group that she first noticed the great differences in the appearance of the women in the class. Always a physically active person, and always concerned with diet and appearance, Susan realized that there must be a lot to learn about aging gracefully. She began to read about preventive healthcare and followed the suggestions that made good sense to her. For example, like most of the coeds of her day, Susan had begun to smoke cigarettes when she was a senior in high school and continued to smoke about a pack of cigarettes a day until she read the Surgeon General's warning issued in 1964. She then stopped smoking.

In 1965, having read Dr. Robert A. Wilson's *Feminine Forever,* which extolled the virtues of the hormone estrogen to maintain youth for menopausal women, she paid close attention and followed all the medical and media hype about hormones throughout the following decade, becoming familiar with the many dissenting medical views on this subject. She watched as women had their high hopes of eternal feminity dashed as more and more medical studies indicated that estrogen caused cancer of the uterus, and perhaps even of the breast. In 1976, physicians drastically reduced their practice of prescribing estrogen.

The current management of menopause by physicians seemed very complicated and inconsistent to Susan, with debate among doctors and researchers alike. Then in 1976, she read of the appointment of a young physician named Wulf Utian to the staff of University Hospitals of Cleveland and to the faculty of Case Western Reserve University School of Medicine. Dr. Utian, she read, was an obstetrician/gynecologist, an M.D. with a Ph.D. in reproductive endocrinology, who had written his doctoral thesis specifically on the treatment of menopause. Earlier in 1967, he had established the first menopause clinic in the world in his native South Africa at the Groote Schuur Hospital. (This institution was renowned for its support of pioneering medical advances; later that same year Dr. Christian Barnard performed the world's first heart transplant there.)

Susan made an appointment with Dr. Utian for a gynecologic physical. Thus, it was at the age of forty-four and in good health that Susan had the opportunity to work with Dr. Utian to preserve and savor as much of her health and youth as possible during her midlife years. After performing a physical examination and a Pap test to check for proper hormone levels and for the presence of cancer cells, Dr. Utian took a holistic approach to Susan's well-being. They discussed at length Susan's diet, her exercise regimen, her reproductive history, and her interest in participating in her own healthcare. They created a complete health plan for Susan that she would follow with Dr. Utian's guidance.

When, at the age of fifty-one, Susan began to experience the early symptoms of menopause—waning and irregular periods and the first hot flashes—she had already been practicing the Utian Menopause Management Program (MMP). Susan went through these years with as little discomfort and as much encouragement as possible and in many ways enhanced her health and appearance through more attention to her diet, a personalized exercise program, hormone replacement therapy, which she chose to take, and the positive attitude, fostered by the MMP, that getting older meant that she was getting better.

We have written this book to put the Utian Menopause Management Program into the hands of women everywhere, providing the tools for living longer and living better, just as Dr. Utian was able to do for Susan. Using the MMP, menopause becomes simply a new stage in the continuing process of life. It is not the final stage.

The Utian Menopause Management Program was developed in the same pioneering spirit with which Dr. Utian first began to do research in the virtually untapped area of menopause. As he recalls,

> I became intrigued by the problems of menopause more than twenty-five years ago. In particular, I was challenged by the physicians' overwhelming lack of concern about the issues facing women whose ovaries had been removed or had failed. I began to study the subject intensely in 1966 and wrote my thesis on the problems of the absent or failing ovary, and how estrogen replacement therapy might help. In doing my research, I was astonished at the insensitive level of care women have endured throughout history. There seemed to be very little real understanding of the events of midlife—and certainly a lack of compassion for the upheaval it caused.

Women's Medicine Comes of Age

Menopause—the cessation of the menses—is a milestone that has been referred to in many early cultures and texts. Initially, an association simply was made between age and the loss of fertility. In the Bible, it is written "God said unto Abraham, as for Sarah thy wife . . . I will bless her and give thee a son also of her . . . then Abraham fell upon his face and said in his heart, shall a child be born unto him that is a hundred years old? And shall Sarah, that is ninety years old bear?'' (Genesis 15:17–18).

By the sixth century A.D., it was well documented that the end of menstruation occurred between the ages of thirty-five and fifty in most women, although one writer of the times stated "Fat women lose their periods very early, and whether the periods remain normal or abnormal, increase in amount or become diminished depends on the age, the season of the year, the habits, the particular traits of women, the nature of foods eaten and complicating diseases." It is interesting that the link between lifestyle and menopause is mentioned here for the first time, but these issues were not actually explored until centuries later.

By 1777, semieducated guesses were made to explain why the menstrual cycle ends; most of them were entirely inaccurate. These early pioneers who studied menstrual function postulated that the cessation of blood flow to the womb caused a woman to appear aged and to become sterile. The literature also reveals that it was thought ridiculous for a woman to consider sexual enjoyment after menopause.

Menopause also became associated with many diseases and was considered to be a negative stage in a woman's life. In 1777, the English gynecologist John Leake wrote in his book, *Chronic or Slow Diseases Peculiar to Women,* that, "At this critical time of life, around age fifty, the female sex are often visited with various diseases of the chronic kind." These included "pain and giddiness of the head, hysteric disorders, colic pains, and a midlife female weakness . . . intolerable itching at the neck of the bladder and contiguous parts are often very troubling." He also noted that, "Women are sometimes affected with low spirits and melancholy." In 1840, British scientist John Burns stated that, "The cessation of menses does of itself seem, in some cases, to excite cancer of the breast." Physicians were flirting with the idea that unusual medical phenomena occurred for many women at the time of menopause, but they continued to comment on the complications rather than search for answers.

In fact, Leake took a reproachful attitude toward women, explaining the discomforts of menopause as caused by the "many excesses introduced by luxury, and the irregularities of the passions." Adding insult to injury, he noted, "Quadrapeds and other animals are entirely exempt [from such diseases] by living comfortable to their natural feelings.''

Laying the blame for menopause on women's excesses continued. In 1868, a French scientist named Charasse wrote that, ''A lady who has during the whole of her wifehood eschewed fashionable society and has lived simply, plainly and sensibly, and who has taken plenty of outdoor exercise, will during the autumn and winter of her life reap her reward by enjoying what is the greatest earthly blessing—health.''

So by the mid- to late nineteenth century, the idea of exercise had been added to the collections of ineptly understood ideas about the effects of diet, sex, stress, and disease on menopausal women. A concrete plan for improving the lives of these women, however, had yet to be formulated. The tendency of these early authors to associate menopause with negative social factors peaked in the mid-nineteenth century when Columbat de L'Isere devoted an entire chapter on the change of life in his *Treatise of the Diseases of Females*. He explained menopause in the following manner:

> Compelled to yield to the power of time, women now cease to exist for the species and henceforward live only for themselves. Their features are stamped with the impress of age and their genital organs are sealed with the signet of sterility. . . . It is the dictate of prudence to avoid all such circumstances as might tend to awaken any erotic thoughts in the mind and reanimate a sentiment that ought rather to become extinct. . . . In fact, everything calculated to cause regret for charms lost and enjoyments that are ended now forever.

Earlier, L'Isere had also stated that ''She now resembles a de-throned queen, or rather a goddess whose adorers no longer frequent her shrine. Should she still retain a few courtiers, she can only attract them by the charm of her wit and the force of her talents.'' With such attitudes prevailing among the ''experts,'' any improvement of the life drama for most women was practically nonexistent.

To be fair, we did discover that a few physicians took a more empathetic attitude toward the plight of women. In 1887, one pioneer, Dr. E. Borner, stated that:

> The climacteric, or so-called change of life in women, presents, without question, one of the most interesting subjects offered to the physician, and especially to the gynecologist in the practice of

his profession. The phenomena of this period are various and changeable, that he must certainly have had a wide experience who has observed and learned to estimate them all. So ill-defined are the boundaries between the physiological and the pathological in this field of study, that it is highly desirable in the interest of our patients of the other sex, that the greatest possible light should be thrown upon this question.

Even with this need noted, it took remarkably long for Borner's call to research to be answered. Not much changed over the many decades that followed. As recently as 1963, prominent physicians R. A. Wilson and T. A. Wilson wrote that, "A large percentage of women . . . acquire a vapid cowlike feeling called a 'negative state.' . . . It is a strange endogenous misery . . . the world appears as through a gray veil and they live as docile, harmless creatures, missing most of life's values."

The significance of menopause finally began to be recognized in 1967. Although it was still described as a tragedy, it was seen as one that should be taken seriously by doctors. Dr. Phillip Rhoades concluded, "Many women are leading an active and productive life when this tragedy strikes. They remain attractive and mentally alert. They deeply resent, what to them, is a catastrophic attack upon their ability to earn a living and to enjoy life."

Only in the second half of the twentieth century has medical interest in improving the second half of women's lives become aroused, with the number of research studies concerning menopause steadily growing. Perhaps this interest reflects the demands of "baby boomers" who are entering midlife, as well as general concern about the growing percentage of the older female population, because paralleling our increasing knowledge about menopause is what the sociologists are calling the "graying of America."

In the United States alone, the population over the age of thirty-five increased 35 percent in 1987 and is projected to continue to expand so swiftly that it will double from the 60 million counted in 1950 to 120 million by 1990. Add to that staggering escalation the fact that a full one-third of the population will be more than fifty years of age within the next decade and it becomes apparent that we must identify midlife health-risk factors earlier and create preventive healthcare programs to meet this growing need. Otherwise, the increased cost of medical care for this greater number of individuals will be foisted upon an already dangerously overburdened medical industry, crippling the healthcare delivery system itself—very likely to the detriment of the women needing it most.

The indications are clear: The older population will be larger, live longer, and will be comprised predominantly of women. Menopause also correlates frequently with an increase in the incidence of diseases such as osteoporosis and coronary heart disease, subjects of great importance to women at midlife. These will be addressed in chapter 3, along with suggestions of ways to minimize your risks.

Another trend over the past fifty years is the increasing incidence of surgical procedures performed on women over the age of thirty-five. The most frequently performed procedure for women is total abdominal hysterectomy, which in too many cases includes the removal of the ovaries. Thus, there will be many more women living much longer without their ovaries. They will be thrust into premature menopause, which deeply affects women's health in ways that will be fully discussed in chapter 3. Unnecessary hysterectomy also increases a woman's risk for developing heart disease and osteoporosis. The situation is alarming!

There is an economic angle to the Utian Menopause Management Program, too. Between 1980 and 1985, health expenditures in the United States jumped from 9.1 percent to 10.7 percent of the gross national product, an increase of almost $700 per person, with 3.5 million more persons enrolled in Medicare. The establishment of preventive health education and evaluation programs for women, as well as women's involvement in programs such as the Utian Menopause Management Program, could help to reverse these healthcare spending trends. All of the preventive health maintenance aspects of the Utian Program, which we will outline in chapter 2, including such things as changes in diet, incorporation of a special exercise program, hormone replacement therapy when appropriate, and daily calcium supplementation, can help women save themselves and the country's insurance programs thousands of dollars in unnecessary diagnoses and procedures.

It is each woman's right and responsibility to initiate preventive healthcare for herself. Our purpose in *Managing Your Menopause* is to provide you with the complete MMP to enable you to do just that. We outline the program in the next chapter, and fill in that outline with easy-to-follow, healthful information throughout the rest of the book. We want to help you maximize the quality of your life! So read on, and take the first step toward a new level of control over your health and your future.

·2·

The Utian Menopause
Management Program

What Is the Utian Menopause
Management Program?

The Utian Menopause Management Program is a new way for you to care for *you.* It is a plan to help you assure your own best passage through midlife and the postmenopausal years. It offers a concrete plan for you to follow within the framework of your own goals for your future. The program is comprised of three crucial components:

1. The latest facts about midlife and health, along with a philosophy, a purpose, and a direction for the second half of your life.
2. Specific tools for you to use to achieve these health goals.
3. Specific action plans to ensure success.

These three components, used successfully for years by Dr. Utian with his patients, will help you toward a longer, healthier, and more fulfilling life, as it has hundreds of other women.

The Twelve Basic Principles of the Utian Program

1. *You can live better and longer.* Statistics show unequivocally that modifying patterns of behavior and practicing appropriate preventive care measures can prolong your life.
2. *Illness and disability are not inevitable in the later years.* There is no doubt that any individual can acquire an unexpected disease that may alter or even shorten her life. However, the majority of major

illnesses have some additional causative factors that relate to personal lifestyle and habits. If you change these, you are working toward a healthier and longer life.

3. *It is within your power to be healthy and vibrant.* Obesity, high blood pressure, heart disease, and osteoporosis are just a few examples of the major illnesses that can be prevented to a large extent by gradual changes in your lifestyle and habits.

4. *You are important, you are wanted, and you are needed.* This principle is one of the most important on which to reflect as you read this book. Many women question their own value and, in so doing, have fallen into one of the worst of the midlife traps: that of putting themselves down and undermining their self-esteem. It is value of yourself that promotes good self-care habits. Positive attitudes create positive behaviors that protect your personal and considerable worth. You will have the opportunity to ponder this idea at important points throughout the book.

5. *Appreciate your additional experience.* Take a new view about the years you have lived. You have gained an appreciable amount of experience. Draw on it. Use your experience to deal more efficiently and effectively with problems and reduce stress in your home, business, and social life. This book will help to show you how.

6. *Repay your debt to yourself.* To most women, the years between the ages of twenty-five and forty-five are an endless stream of devotion of life, effort, and spirit to their families, to jobs, to aging parents, or to any combination of these factors. Few of us escape the personal responsibilities that are a part of the richness of life. All too often, however, family members and colleagues take as their right what you have given as their privilege: your loyalty and your loving care. By the age of menopause, your children are grown and close to or fully independent, and your mate is at the peak of his career and maybe even beginning to relax a little. Now is the time for you to take stock of yourself. What is actually happening in your own life? Have you given all of yourself to everyone but yourself? What do you owe *you?*

Now is the time when you must realize that to keep yourself operating in high gear, you owe yourself something special. Do not confuse this principle with selfishness; it is not. It is consideration of self. You deserve to give yourself the time and the effort necessary to improve the quality of the rest of your life.

7. *You are as old as you allow yourself to feel.* Many clichés are true and perhaps none is more true than the statement that you are only

as old as you feel. Despite health problems, some chronically ill people impress everyone with their joy of life. Many elderly people, healthy or not, are great company. They continue to attract people as they always did. They speak with enthusiasm of the present and the future. Other people whom you know may be younger in years, but they think old, talk old, and, as a result, feel old. Age is not the determinant factor here—attitude is, and it is adjustable. Therefore, you can stop feeling old by understanding that you are only as old as you let yourself feel.

8. *Time flies—each day really is a once-in-a-lifetime opportunity.* Many people view the swift passage of time as a negative idea. This type of thinking is contrary to living a productive and satisfying life. You can view time from a positive perspective: It must be made the most of through effective and efficient usage. Do not waste it! Use every day to its fullest!

9. *If you have money, spend it on yourself.* Many parents feel uncomfortable when they are advised to spend time and money on themselves. They are so accustomed to worrying about the family and the children that they see personal use of funds as diminishing inheritance for their children. Utter nonsense! If you have children, you have reared them to be independent; let them rely on themselves. Any legacy from you, then, becomes a bonus. At this time of your life, you must plan for your own secure and comfortable retirement. Extra benefits derived from extra funds are *your* bonus.

10. *Ignore societal attitudes that are outdated.* Virtually all negative attitudes toward menopause within our society are fallacies based on tradition and superstition. Ignore them in terms of your lifestyle and discredit them by your actions. Consider using your influence within the community to change attitudes toward women at midlife, particularly through the media, where women have not been reflected in a positive way.

11. *Enjoyment of life is not sinful or self-indulgent.* Have fun! Whenever appropriate and wherever you can, enjoy yourself. The benefits of a positive and playful attitude will show in your demeanor and even in your appearance. Having fun is contagious, too. It will have a tonic effect on your relationships and on how others see you and respond to you.

12. *You can control your destiny.* Your attitude and your actions can, in many respects, determine the success or failure of your life. If you view your midlife years as negative ones, they probably will fulfill

your prophecy. On the other hand, if you fill these years with satisfying projects, they will be a time of reduced stress and increased pleasure.

These are the dozen principles that serve as the foundation of the Utian Program. They can be learned, practiced, and incorporated into your lifestyle using the tools described below.

The Eight Essential Tools of the Utian Program

1. *You, yourself.* You may have a difficult time viewing yourself as a tool. However, it is important to understand that the first major resource of the program that you have to work with is *you.* You will learn how to view yourself this way as you carry out the Utian Program.

2. *A physician whom you trust and respect.* Medical advice and care are also tools to be used, and your physician is the number one tool in your armamentarium. Although he or she cannot deliver miracles, do take advantage of the modern medical treatments available and the sound advice provided by a solid continuing relationship with an interested physician. Chapter 3 reveals how you can become an active participant with your physician in planning your health programs.

3. *Hormone treatment may work for you.* Hormone treatment is not the number one tool because it is not the only tool and it is not for all women. Hormones also do not work all by themselves to create a first-rate second half of life. They are *one method* of ensuring good health following menopause. They are extremely important but cannot be considered of value when they are utilized alone. Hormone replacement therapy and nonhormonal therapy will be described in chapter 5, and the risks and benefits of hormone treatment will be fully explored in chapter 6.

4. *The right diet.* Common sense should reign when it comes to diet, but it doesn't always. Although you know that a nutritious, well-balanced diet is important, if you are like most people, you probably take certain shortcuts and may be over- or underweight. In either case, the Utian Program will help you change your eating patterns and create a permanent and appropriate diet. Being overweight causes a multiplicity of disadvantages to your health and lon-

gevity as well as to your appearance and comfort. The same is true of being underweight, because women who are too thin shrink their prospects for a healthy and long life just as they shrink their bodies.

The Utian Menopause Dietstyle, described in detail in chapter 7 of this book, is nutritionally sound for women who are underweight, overweight, or who are at their goal weight. It includes all the food groups, minerals, and vitamins that are essential for women's lifelong health and well-being.

5. *Exercise that makes you feel and look great.* Women at midlife who have always exercised are in the best shape for continued and appropriate physical activity. Women who have exercised minimally or who have been sedentary can use the Utian Program to incorporate exercise easily into their lives. There are some important exercise do's and don'ts for women at midlife. Designed in cooperation with exercise physiologists and the most current philosophy of physical activity, chapter 8 outlines the best exercise options for the midlife woman. We will describe in detail different types of exercise that promote heart and lung fitness, work toward the prevention of osteoporosis, and even enhance your sex life.

6. *Total body care.* The care that you devote to your body has a direct effect on your feelings. You know that how you *think* you look directly affects how you *feel.* It also affects how others feel about you, which has a reciprocal effect on all of your valued interpersonal relationships. Judicious and proper use of cosmetics, and the care you give your skin and your hair, can enhance your appearance. These things are most important now when you cannot rely simply on the scrubbed face of youth as your ally.

The Utian Program offers valuable guidelines on all aspects of how you care for you. These pointers are carefully chosen and discussed because they ensure that you are maximizing the health of all your body parts, from teeth to toes. The care of your hair is important, too, because it will last and shine with your special care and will befriend your appearance if you give it the time and the style that it requires. The glow of health can be achieved with special care of the skin, particularly of the face, neck, and décolletage. Cosmetics, carefully selected and judiciously used, can enhance this effect. Tips for selecting and using skin care and cosmetic products will be described in chapter 11, as will special care for the hands and the nails.

You can't look good on the outside unless you feel good on the inside. We will provide information on how to make the most of regular medical checkups as well as which medical tests should be performed, when, and why at midlife and beyond.

7. *Wearing the clothes that suit you.* Correct dress is very important, especially as a woman enters midlife. You should dress for the role you have decided to play—business executive to bohemian—but make sure that you do not miscast yourself. Take time to notice what looks good on you. If you still have the figure for tight blue jeans and you prefer them, wear them; but avoid extremes. Hems go up and hems go down in length, but the only aspect of that yo-yo that is important is that you go to all kinds of lengths to wear only what looks good on you. The appearance you present helps to shape how people interact with you.

8. *Finding menopause clinics and support groups.* If you benefit from group support and encouragement, seek it out! Your physician or local hospital should be able to direct you to a menopause support group in your area. If not, why not be the initiator yourself and get such a group started? Our experience has shown that there are many, many women going through the menopause experience who would welcome the opportunity to learn from and share with other women. The address of the North American Menopause Society is listed in appendix D. A letter to the society will bring you the most current information about existing facilities, menopause clinics, and support groups in your area. The society can also provide guidance for setting up a support group if none is available in your area.

Now that you know about the eight tools available to you through the Utian Menopause Management Program, let's look at the techniques for using them effectively.

Getting Started with the Utian Method

Take an impartial look at yourself. First, find a full-length mirror. Stand in front of it and take an impartial look at yourself. Be critical, but also be *fair* to yourself, and be honest. Do you like what you see? If you were sitting at a sidewalk café on the Left Bank in Paris in April and you saw yourself go by, would you want to know more about that person? What comments might you make to your companion? "There goes someone who cares for herself and takes care of herself." Or would you see yourself as someone who has lost interest in herself and in life? Are you someone you would like to know?

If you like what you see, then you undoubtedly still have that important zest for life. This program will enhance that sparkle in your eye! If you see room for improvement, take a deep breath and congratulate yourself. You have just taken the first step toward a new you—by being willing to be honest about your life today.

Imagine yourself as you would like to be. If you are not satisfied with your mirror image, visualize the you that *you* would like to see. Carefully consider and list the factors at fault. Weight? Posture? Hair? Skin? Cosmetics? Clothing? Each of these can be corrected with a little personal loving care.

Now imagine yourself slimmer and trimmer, standing taller, with a new and appropriate hairdo, properly applied cosmetics, a new style of dress that brings out your best, and a smile on your face. If you prefer that new image, then make it your objective to attain it.

Use your tools. The tools listed earlier in this chapter are designed with the new you in mind. Use each tool now to your advantage. Your objective is inner and outer health.

Consider yourself first. Remember that you are important, you are wanted, and you are needed. Decide to live each day to its fullest. Plan ahead for positive experiences. Take ten minutes today to plan a nice "something" for yourself tomorrow. Become motivated about caring for yourself and be enthusiastic about yourself, your family, and your friends. Enthusiasm is contagious. You will be continually surprised, and sometimes amazed, at how your new positive attitude affects your family and your friends in a favorable way.

Warn your man. If there is a man in your life, warn him that you are adopting the Utian Program's suggested methods for self-improvement. Tell him that this program is how you have determined to sail through midlife and beyond, and elicit his support and companionship in your quest to savor each day and each experience.

Play your role right. Whatever image you have decided you prefer for yourself must become the role you are now going to play. Whether it is mature professional or senior tennis champion, the life of the party or the intellectual, a devotee of the arts or a long-distance walker, play it to the hilt. This is not a recommendation for deception of self or others, but you must make a total commitment in order to build a solid self-image and fulfill it. Obviously, you want your objective to be reasonable and attainable. So select from within your own storehouse of accomplishments those you wish to pursue with added gusto and zest.

Get involved. Once you have decided your personal role, carefully define that role within your immediate family, within your circle of close friends, within your community, and in regard to your future in society. Be thankful for what you have and for the spare time that you have finally realized. Your children are independent, your mate is settled in his pursuits, and you are settled in yours. Perhaps for the first time, you have some free time. Relish it and use it wisely.

If charitable work interests you, find a worthy cause that is particularly meaningful to you and give of your time and yourself. If you have always been politically inclined, seek public office locally or nationally. Was your earlier professional or technical training interrupted by raising a family? Consider refresher courses at college and go back to work. For many women, the pride of self-fulfillment, with or without the independence of monetary reward, coupled with the joy of being deeply involved in worthwhile pursuits, is a boost to self-confidence.

If you love social activities, they are rewarding as well. Learn to play bridge, tennis, or golf. Take up dancing or bowling. If you are drawn to the arts, then learn to paint, write, sculpt, pot, make jewelry, or refinish furniture. Or create the lushest, most unusual, most fruitful garden!

The activity you choose is not important. The fact that you are busy with something you enjoy is vital. If you are not getting involved at midlife, when *will* you get involved?

Get up and go. This is our foremost wish for you. It's time to revalue yourself. Like all things of value, you have appreciated with age. Appreciate that fact! Reestablish all your important connections and make new ones as well. Keep active. It will keep you looking and feeling young.

Only you can create an even better life after menopause by becoming fully informed about your options and by taking positive action. Using the program outlined in this book, you can take charge of the second half of your life with zest, commitment, and joy!

·3·

Finding Dr. Right

Menopause is an event common to all women. For some women, it is not difficult, but for many it arrives with complications, both physiological and psychological.

Today, a healthy fifty-year-old woman can reasonably expect to live for another thirty to forty years. Doctors are now becoming more aware of the need to help women turn these postmenopausal years into quality years.

In an ideal scenario, long before menopause, each woman would have found her ideal physician. Over the years, she would have been able to sit for hours with her doctor and acquaint him or her with all the details relevant to her medical history. She would visit the doctor with a complete list of pertinent questions and the doctor would have all the right answers and take the time to share them with her.

Yet, how many women actually have this experience? Very few. One reason is because the medical care for women at midlife has been so haphazard. Physicians are only now beginning to understand the female climacteric—that ten-year transitional period surrounding menopause. Perhaps many women feel that they are lucky if they can get through menopause, by themselves, without seeking the often complicating and shifting views of doctors.

What Midlife Means to You

So much happens in your life when you are approaching and experiencing the years that surround that milestone—menopause—that occurs around the age of fifty. Your work life may be gearing up or down. Your children may marry and leave home. You may have to handle your parents' illnesses or death. You may become a grandmother for the first time. You will also experience menopause. It is apparent that an incredible amount of change will be going on in your life.

In an effort to learn how women view menopause, the International Health Foundation surveyed four hundred women in each of five countries: Belgium, France, Great Britain, Italy, and West Germany—a total of two thousand postmenopausal women. The results of the 1970 survey concluded that for many women, menopause is a period of disorientation, physical discomfort, and emotional upheaval. The postmenopausal period was described as a time when women could not feel as content as they had in their premenopausal state. Further, the survey revealed that menopause is more difficult for women who lack the social supports that more affluent women have available to them. Women who engaged in activities such as those described in my program seemed to bounce back better from "the menopause crisis," as the study termed it.

I want to assure you that menopause is not a "crisis." It is, however, a transitional process that occurs on social, emotional, and medical levels. To make menopause a comfortable transition, I believe that doctors must offer preventive medical programs to women over the age of forty-five that prevent estrogen deficiency and its subsequent medical and psychological problems, as well as offer a way to affirm productive attitudes and actions for midlife women.

Today, nearly twenty years after the International Health Foundation's survey, women still are not sure what to do about menopause. A 1987 Harris Survey showed that American women are confused and misinformed about menopause and its treatment. The survey results were compiled following telephone interviews with five hundred women between the ages of forty-five and seventy, evenly divided among ten major U.S. cities: Boston, New York, Washington, Atlanta, Seattle, Los Angeles, Phoenix, Chicago, Memphis, and Houston. These are all cities in which the best of American medicine is provided. The interviews covered the subject of menopause, its treatment, its symptoms, and other related women's health issues. Sixty percent of the interviewees were postmenopausal, 22 percent were experiencing menopause, and 16 percent were premenopausal.

The dismal findings indicated that a very small percentage of the women knew the long-term consequences of estrogen deficiency.

Fewer than half of the study participants could name a single treatment for the common menopausal symptoms that affect more than 85 percent of all women at menopause such as night sweats, vaginal dryness, and hot flashes.

Although this menopause survey drew similar responses throughout the country, there were some interesting regional differences. For example, the highest level of confusion about effective treatment of menopausal symptoms was in the Southeast, where a significant number of women mistakenly believed that antidepressants, aspirin, and tranquilizers were effective therapy. The Northeast registered the highest number of women who were unable to name any form of treatment. Just 40 percent of the women in the West knew about the role of the ovaries and estrogens in preventing osteoporosis—a serious degenerative condition of the bone that afflicts women—which made them the most knowledgeable group about hormone replacement therapy in the country!

These survey results reflect a high level of confusion among women about menopause. How can a woman get the medical help she needs if she is not informed about what is happening to her, what to expect, and how to get help when help is needed?

Below is a list of questions most commonly asked by my patients. You may find them useful in talking with your own doctor, and in evaluating the medical information you are given.

The Q and A of Menopause

Q. What is menopause?
A. Menopause is a milestone marking your last menstrual period and the transition from the reproductive to the nonreproductive time of life. For some women it is a smooth transition; for others it creates both physiological and psychological discomforts.

Among doctors, the crucial question about menopause has always been whether it represents a normal developmental stage in a woman's life cycle or whether it is a hormone deficiency syndrome related to the failure of the ovary, requiring diagnosis and treatment.

I believe that menopause is a normal and significant point in a woman's life cycle that may be associated with some uncomfortable symptoms and, sometimes, with the risk of more serious illness. Menopause happens to all women, but affects each one uniquely. The good news that we want to share in this book is that it is possible to prevent most of the more severe effects of menopause.

Q. What do I need to know about midlife and menopause?

A. Since the first step in prevention is understanding, let's start with a brief overview of the most important points to remember about the fascinating systems that operate in women's lives.

The human body is an exquisite mechanism constructed so that each system works in a delicate balance with other processes within the body. This idea of balance and interrelationship is especially important in understanding what occurs at midlife.

Your monthly cycle is controlled by certain centers in your brain. They signal appropriate body parts and systems, "telling" them when and how to operate. The description below figure 1 should clarify this process.

Often women ask me whether they have a glandular problem. It is important to understand just how the glands work within your cycle. There are two types of glands in the body: *exocrine* and *endocrine.* The *exocrine glands* release chemical substances directly to the area where they are needed. A good example is the sweat glands, which aid in the cooling of the skin, and the sebaceous glands, which secrete oils that keep the skin pliable. When menopause arrives, these glands may not work as effectively because of the changes in their "programming." The sweat glands may not "cool" as efficiently and the sebaceous glands may not keep the skin as soft and smooth as before. *Endocrine glands,* in contrast, produce and release their substances directly into the bloodstream. These substances are chemical messengers called *hormones.*

Before menopause, your monthly cycle is under the control of certain centers in the brain. The brain is our ultimate computer, handling billions of messages, signals, and functions, all operating simultaneously with remarkable order and purpose. *Neurotransmitters* are the "messengers" that activate the appropriate brain areas and systems, "telling" them when to go into operation, or when to alter their function.

Brain activity is controlled by messages from both inside and outside of the body. It is within the *cerebral cortex,* or higher brain

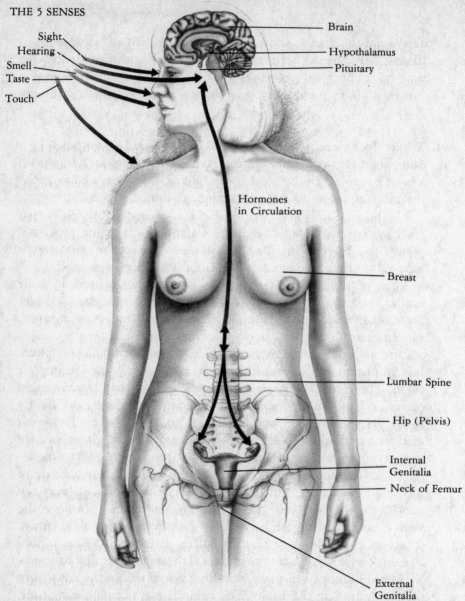

Figure 1. Interaction of Senses and Hormones.
Chemical messages are interpreted within the brain, triggering chemical signals that are to be sent throughout the body. The ovary reacts and, in turn, sends the messages to body tissues and back to the brain. Stimuli from the outside, via the senses, may also influence these interactions.

areas, that we are made aware of ourselves, our surroundings, and our sense of well-being. When signals go awry in this area of the brain, the results are changed emotions, feelings, and perceptions.

Tucked in the base of the brain in the middle of the skull lies the funnel-shaped *hypothalamus,* one of our most important endocrine glands. It is to the human body what mission control is to space flight. Messages or impulses from our senses, such as sight, smell, hearing, taste, and touch, are eventually directed to the hypothalamus, which is strategically connected to all other areas of the brain. You can follow its route in figure 1.

The hypothalamus produces several hormones, but the one that is of importance in understanding the female monthly cycle is called the *gonadotropin releasing hormone* (GRH). GRH dictates action in another important gland, the *pituitary,* a pea-sized structure lying directly beneath the hypothalamus in a bony cave at the base of the skull. The pituitary, in turn, produces the hormones that control, amongst other glands, the all-powerful *ovary.* The pituitary secretes two hormones called the *gonadotropins:* individually called the *follicle stimulating hormone* (FSH) and the *luteinizing hormone* (LH). These are the hormones that directly affect the growth and development of the ovarian follicle. The FSH stimulates the follicle to ripen and the LH matures the egg and causes its release.

The ovary is the most powerful gland in a woman's body, producing those two sex hormones, *estrogen* and *progesterone,* that make the differences between men and women. Women have two ovaries that have two directly interrelated functions: to produce those sex hormones and to produce eggs.

Before a female child is born, there are probably several million eggs in her ovaries, but for unknown reasons, this number reduces to about 500,000 eggs at her birth. Unlike the male, who is able to produce new spermatozoa for the rest of his life, the female ovary can only lose eggs until the supply is depleted at menopause. The supply of eggs is actually programed for exhaustion. The ovary raises hundreds of follicles each month, each containing an egg, but only one egg is expelled in the menstrual cycle (except in the rare case of multiple fraternal births). The others are lost. In figure 2, you can see a cross section of the ovary before and after menopause. Notice the differences.

Almost every part of your body is changed somewhat by the

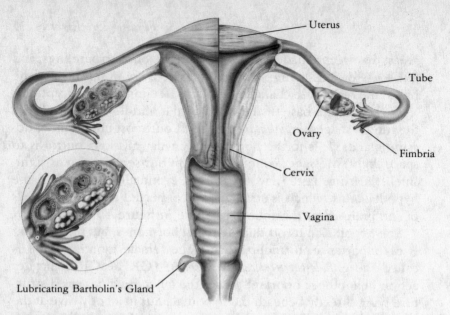

Uterus

Tube

Ovary

Fimbria

Cervix

Vagina

Lubricating Bartholin's Gland

BEFORE MENOPAUSE

AFTER MENOPAUSE

Figure 2. Cross-Section of the Internal Genitalia.

Before menopause *(left):* The detail of the ovary shows the development cycle of an egg starting with the early graafian follicle, release of the egg into the fallopian tube, and the conversion of the follicle into the corpus luteum and corpus albicans.

After menopause *(right):* The tissues after menopause clearly show the thinning and shrinking resulting from decreased ovarian hormone production.

levels of estrogen and progesterone your ovary is producing. *All* of the sex organs, both inside and outside of the body, need estrogen in order to work properly. Figure 3 demonstrates the differences in the external sex organs when estrogen is lacking. Notice the reduced size of the clitoris and outer labia and the loss of pubic hair. Changes also occur inside the body as the walls of the vagina and the uterus gradually become thinner without estrogen. Refer again to figure 2 to view the effects of estrogen deprivation. The diagram in figure 4 shows where certain other important pelvic organs are located in relation to the sex organs. The bladder lies just in front of the uterus. The tube through which the bladder empties, the urethra, lies in front of the vagina. The bowel is behind the uterus, and the rectum and the opening of the bowel, the anus, are behind the vagina. This diagram will be useful for reference as we review other changes. As you will see in chapter 6, the relationship of all these organs to the vagina is of importance when we consider the problem of *prolapse,* or drop, of the pelvic organs, a condition that often becomes a problem in the early postmenopausal years.

The female *breast,* figure 5, has been idolized and romanticized in poetry and prose throughout history. Although this organ has miraculous capabilities, it is important to remember that the functions of the breast are not related to their size or shape. Breasts are comprised of glandular tissue surrounded by fat, which serves as a kind of packing tissue. The ducts from the glands end in the nipple. Another important fact to remember about the breast is that these glands react to the presence or absence of hormones and also that the glands are the site for cancer when it develops in the breast.

Many patients ask why breasts droop with age. As you can see in the diagram, fibrous bands known as Cooper's ligaments run throughout the breast and are attached to firm tissue that lies like a sheet covering the chest wall. The stretching of these bands caused by weight, gravity, and aging accounts for breast sag.

Q. What makes menopause occur?

A. Menopause happens when the ovaries run out of eggs or are surgically removed. Let's examine the role of the potent ovary and how it shapes some of the stages in women's lives.

A young girl's reproductive years begin with her first menstrual period, or *menarche.* This monthly cycle continues (unless interrupted by childbirth) until menopause, the final menstrual period. Menopause occurs on average at fifty-one years of age. You recall that the symptoms that may appear around the time of menopause are collectively named the *climacteric,* the period usually between the ages of forty-five and fifty-five. The period of several years before menopause is sometimes referred to as the *perimenopause,* and the years following menopause are called the *postmenopause,* which gradually merges with the *senium,* or old age.

Although these stages occur in all women's lives, each woman can modify some of these stages to her own advantage. Many of the discomforts of menopause can be alleviated by the exciting new advances in science and with preventive programs you can put into practice easily.

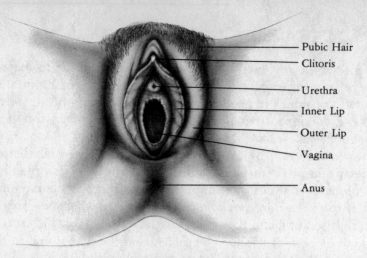

Pubic Hair

Clitoris

Urethra

Inner Lip

Outer Lip

Vagina

Anus

BEFORE MENOPAUSE

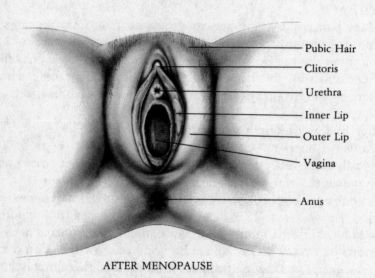

Pubic Hair

Clitoris

Urethra

Inner Lip

Outer Lip

Vagina

Anus

AFTER MENOPAUSE

Figure 3. External Genitalia.
Before menopause *(above).*
    After menopause *(below).*
After menopause, the apparent widening of the vaginal opening is the result of reduced muscle tone in the pelvic organs following reduced estrogen stimulation.

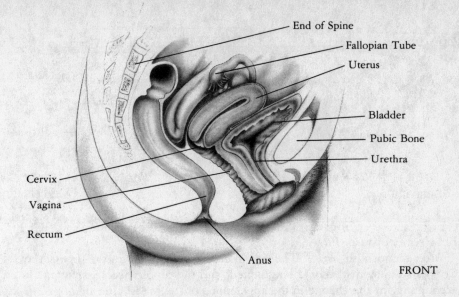

End of Spine
Fallopian Tube
Uterus
Bladder
Pubic Bone
Urethra

Cervix
Vagina
Rectum

Anus

FRONT

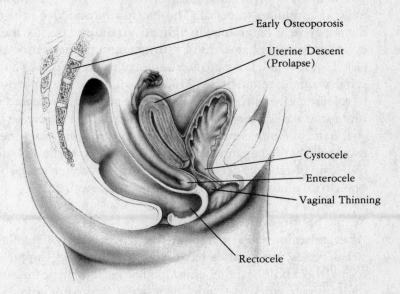

Early Osteoporosis

Uterine Descent
(Prolapse)

Cystocele
Enterocele
Vaginal Thinning

Rectocele

Figure 4. Cross-Section of the Pelvis.
Before menopause *(above):* Cross-section of the pelvis and contents before menopause.

After menopause *(below):* Cross-section of the pelvis and contents after menopause showing the slight dropping of the uterus and prolapse of the bladder and the rectum. Note the narrowing and shortening of the vagina.

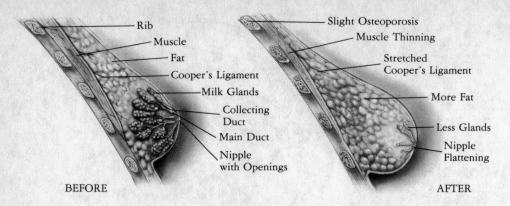

BEFORE   AFTER

Figure 5. Cross-Section of the Breast.
Before menopause *(left)*.

After menopause *(right):* There is increased fat content in the breast, the Cooper's ligaments become lengthened, and the nipple becomes flattened, accounting for the change in the appearance of the breast after menopause.

The ovary controls the reproductive system and, as long as it has eggs, it continues to do so. The entire reproductive, or egg-producing cycle, is diagramed in figure 6. At the end of each menstrual cycle, only a small amount of estrogen and progesterone remains (1). This low level of estrogen and progesterone acts as a thermostat that signals to the brain (2) and tells it to stimulate the ovary (3) to release more estrogen. When more estrogen is released (4) the brain stimulates the ovary again at mid-cycle (5) to release the egg (6). After the egg is released, the ovary adds progesterone to the estrogen that it began releasing continuously earlier in the cycle (7). If no pregnancy occurs, the amount of estrogen and progesterone drops again, starting the menstrual period.

Q. **What happens after menopause?**
A. After releasing eggs for about thirty-five years of regular menstrual cycles, the ovaries have depleted their egg supplies. As a result, the whole system begins to change. The hypothalamus and the pituitary work overtime, producing large amounts of GRH, FSH, and LH, but the aging ovary has depleted its supply of eggs and cannot respond. It is at this point that a woman becomes postmenopausal. The real difference in women after menopause is in the amount of hormone that is produced by the ovaries. It is these changes in hormone levels after menopause that ultimately affect all of your tissues.

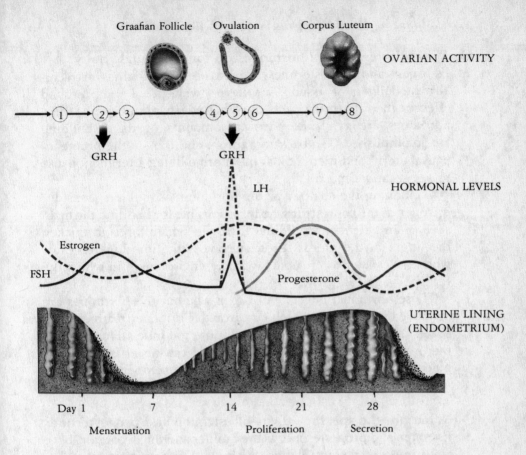

Figure 6. Summary of the Reproductive Cycle: Days 1 to 28.
Low estrogen and progesterone (1) reminds the hypothalamus to produce
GRH (2), which stimulates the pituitary to release FSH (3). This process
stimulates the graafian follicle to grow and make estrogen (4), which rises
to a peak and advises the hypothalamus that it is ripe and ready for the next
step. The hypothalamic surge of GRH (5) passes the message onto the
pituitary, and a surge of LH (6) releases the egg and causes formation of the
corpus luteum. Progesterone and estrogen from the corpus luteum (7) last
fourteen days and then decrease (8) with the formation of the corpus albicans, reminding the hypothalamus to start the whole cycle once again. The
changing estrogen and progesterone levels have a direct effect on the growth
and differentiation of the uterine lining (endometrium) actually preparing it
to receive a fertilized egg.

Q. What do female sex hormones do for the female body?

A. Estrogens and progesterones, the female sex hormones, are actually the builders of tissue. They have a widespread and profound effect on many parts of your body. When adequate amounts of these hormones are available, adequate amounts of tissue building are accomplished. Go back to figure 4 and look at the premenopausal uterus and then look at the uterine lining after menopause to see what we mean.

Continuing the analogy of the hormones as builders, consider estrogen as the contractor who is responsible for building the main shell of an apartment building. Estrogen's main job is to thicken the lining of the uterus. Progesterone is the interior decorator who arrives later to create a favorable environment in which the fertilized egg can grow.

These hormonal effects will occur whether the hormones are produced by the ovary itself or through hormone treatments. In either case, too much estrogen will cause too much thickening of the uterine lining, or endometrium, and can result in abnormal bleeding patterns. This fact is important to remember in undertaking hormone therapy after menopause, the subject of chapter 5.

Q. What are the specific effects of estrogen and progesterone?

A. Estrogen and progesterone, as the builder and the decorator, have many important effects all over the body. You can appreciate these effects best by learning what changes after menopause. When these hormones are not present, the effects that they had on pelvic tissues are lost as well. The table on page 39 shows the various symptoms that can affect the body when it lacks these hormones. We will describe how you can enhance your chances of avoiding most of these problems in chapter 5, so read on with that positive idea in mind.

Let's examine in more detail what happens to the body when it begins to run out of estrogen and progesterone.

Vulva and Vagina

Over the years, sexual intercourse, pregnancy, and childbirth produce a number of changes in the vulva. Stretching or tearing of the perineum, the area between the vagina and the anus, may shorten it, making the vaginal orifice appear wider and more exposed to outside infection. After menopause, the vulval structures gradually undergo shrinkage, which may cause loss of sensation and painful intercourse. Pubic hair is progressively lost, and the skin in that area becomes thinner. In old age it may have a glazed or shiny appearance. The subcutaneous tissues begin to disappear until the labia majora, or outer lips, of the vagina become very small and the labia minora, or inner lips, become almost nonexistent. Postmenopausal women often notice skin changes and itching of the vulva, but no reliable data confirm a direct relationship between those changes and a lack of hormones.

When the hormone estrogen is present, the vulva and the vagina experience cell growth and their pH factor (level of acidity) remains fairly constant. During and following menopause, because of the decrease in hormone and a resulting change in acidity, the vagina may become inflamed or irritated. The vaginal wall becomes shorter and narrower. These changes may make a woman more susceptible to infection as well as cause painful intercourse, which may be helped by using lubricating jellies. It is important to note that although many of these changes are hormone dependent, some of them may be prevented or slowed down considerably by having intercourse regularly. This possibility may be due to the "use it or lose it" theory, which proposes that stimulation on a regular basis may itself prevent dryness. It is even theorized that the absorption of hormones from a partner's ejaculate may be beneficial.

Uterus

Alterations in menstrual patterns and the eventual cessation of periods is the first overt evidence of the climacteric. After menopause, the uterus becomes smaller and its walls become thinner. The *endometrium* (the mucous lining of the uterus), however, can still respond to estrogen if it is provided, changing in thickness and structure as it did with the phases of the menstrual cycle. The relationship between the growth of cells in the endometrium and constantly elevated estrogen levels in the blood is an important one when the subject of cancer of the uterus is discussed later in this book.

Fallopian Tubes

After menopause the fallopian tubes simply cease to function, since no eggs are traveling through them toward the uterus. This stoppage has virtually no effect on women.

Pelvic Floor

Changes in the pelvic floor, that muscular basinlike structure at the base of the pelvis, may occur with pregnancy, when it can become stretched or damaged. During the climacteric, when the ovary begins to produce less estrogen, this muscular tissue becomes more flaccid. The loss of estrogen coupled with the aging of the tissue itself accounts for an increase in problems such as *cystocele,* a protrusion of the urinary bladder through the vaginal wall; *rectocele,* a protrusion of the rectum into the vagina; or *enterocele,* a herniation of the intestine into the vagina. The problem of uterine prolapse, or dropping, and any combination of these conditions may occur and may require surgical correction.

Bladder and Urethra

Postmenopausal changes in the bladder can create some of the most uncomfortable problems for women. Women frequently have repeated bouts with bladder infections. Stress incontinence, or the inability to refrain from discharging urine under stresses, such as jogging, running, sneezing, or even laughing, may occur. Another annoying symptom may be the frequent need to urinate even though the bladder is empty. There is, however, reason to believe that the steadily dropping hormone levels create these problems. The reasons for these changes will be discussed more fully in chapter 5. Estrogen therapy may result in a lessening or disappearance of urinary infection, incontinence, and urgency.

Q. **Are there any other effects of hormone loss?**
A. There are widespread effects upon other organs and tissues of the body caused by menopause or by surgical removal of both ovaries at any age. Researchers are still learning about the effect of menopause upon other areas of the body, but, at present, the following issues are the most important.

Neuroendocrinological Symptoms

The *hot flash* or *hot flush* is the most common and characteristic symptom of the climacteric. For some women, it may be the earliest and also the most troublesome of symptoms. There really is a difference between the flash and the flush. Clinically, the flash precedes the flush and is actually the warning signal that lets you know that you are about to experience a flush.

Although many studies have been done, none has revealed the

exact cause of this bothersome symptom nor have they been able to clarify why some women have flushes and others do not, or why hot flushes persist for years in some women whereas in others they last for only a few months. What we do know, however, is that when estrogen production drops abruptly during the perimenopause, there is a change in the brain's chemistry that affects the temperature control center in the hypothalamus. The result is a decrease in the body's core temperature set point that triggers dilation of the blood vessels of the skin and sweating as the body attempts to reset its thermostat. This process is characteristic of the flush. Other changes in the endocrine system may also influence the symptom of hot flushes, but more studies must be done. Methods for treating hot flushes successfully will be described in chapter 5.

Breasts

The breasts are affected significantly by menopause and by the surgical removal of the ovaries. Each month, during the normal reproductive cycle, your breasts change. Hormones influence glandular formation so that in the first half of the cycle your breasts are less full, and in the second half of the menstrual cycle a combination of glandular proliferation and water retention can increase breast size. These changes cause the symptoms normally described during the menstrual cycle as fullness or tenderness.

After menopause, the glandular tissue of the breast becomes atrophic, or shrinks. Breasts of thin women often become smaller and flatter; those in obese women can remain large and become pendulous. The breasts will also become atrophic rather quickly after surgical menopause, changing in as little as six months after removal of functional ovaries from premenopausal women. The loss of elasticity in the Cooper's ligament aggravates the tendency of the breasts to droop and the nipples become smaller and flatter and may lose their erectile properties.

Thyroid Function

Thyroid changes may occur with age, but there does not appear to be a link between a change in thyroid function and menopause. This fact is hard to explain because increased estrogen is known to have a profound effect on thyroid function tests. It still may be worthwhile for your physician to check your thyroid when examining you in midlife.

Skeleton

A friend of mine was asked by his son why grandmothers always have to be so small. This youngster was making an interesting observation. Did your mother grow shorter as she aged? Have you seen an older woman struggling to carry her parcels from the supermarket, or struggling just to climb stairs? None of that has to happen to you. It all has to do with the skeleton, the bony frame we depend on for support.

Our skeleton is made of living tissue. It does not at all resemble the static steel supports of a building or the chassis of an automobile, yet it has an even more important job of support to do. Fortunately for humans, there is a constant process of adding material to and removing material from the skeleton. This process is called *bone remodeling.* To serve us well, our skeleton requires a delicate balance of addition and subtraction. When more bone is removed than is added to the skeleton, we lose bone mass. Severe loss of bone becomes a condition of brittle bones called *osteoporosis,* which is not a disease but a symptom showing that there has been a loss of the strength of the bone because of a loss in bone mass.

Loss of bone mass becomes a problem when the thinned bone encounters a stress that can break or fracture it. It may take a major impact or hard fall, but sometimes just the jarring of your body caused when your car hits a bump in the road can be enough to injure the driver or the passenger with osteoporosis, causing compression of the vertebrae so that they flatten slightly and actually change the shape of the spine, weakening it. Similarly, just stepping off the curb or suffering a slight jolt could be sufficient stress to fracture a bone.

Osteoporosis has been called "the silent thief," working overtime to rob the skeleton of bone and women of quality of life. More than half of the 40 million American women fifty years of age or older are likely to have detectable changes in their spines. More than one-third of them will eventually have major orthopedic problems caused by osteoporosis.

Postmenopausal osteoporosis is the culprit in the more than 250,-000 hip fractures that occur in the United States each year. These fractures cost 10 billion dollars per year; the human toll is far greater. Half of the women who suffer hip fractures are unable to resume independent existence, with one-fourth of them requiring continuous care in nursing institutions. About 10 percent of these women will die within the first year following the fracture from the complications of associated diseases, such as pneumonia and blood clots that travel to the lungs.

You can avoid this devastating illness. We know most of the causes of osteoporosis, and this crippling condition is preventable as long as you begin and stick with a preventive program.

Preventing Bone Loss. Whether or not you will suffer with this problem is determined by how well your body balances its bone remodeling. In the process of bone remodeling during the first thirty-five to forty years of your life, provided your general health and nutrition are normal, you will deposit more bone than you lose. As a result, your skeleton will enlarge and become stronger and you will reach your *peak bone mass* (the most bone you will ever have) sometime in your mid- to late thirties. Generally, women have less bone mass than men, and go into the second half of their lives with that relative disadvantage. The extent of your peak bone mass and the rate at which you lose bone will determine your bone health in midlife and beyond.

The first several years following menopause are characterized in some women by a phase called *rapid bone loss,* caused by loss of ovarian function. If, over time, the remodeling process continues to be out of balance so that you lose more bone than you deposit, osteoporosis could result. Exercise, diet, and calcium supplementation can help to stabilize the remodeling process and will be discussed in chapters 7 and 8.

Remember that starting around age forty, both men and women lose bone as they age, but women lose more bone at a faster rate because of menopause. Within a few years after menopause, the rate of bone loss slows down, but by that time some women could be in trouble because they started with less bone than men. If you add women's longer life expectancy to this imbalance, you can see how osteoporosis can become a serious concern.

Risk Factors in Osteoporosis. Your chances of developing osteoporosis are higher if you are white or Oriental, if you had your ovaries removed before menopause or had an early menopause, or if you smoke or abuse alcohol. They are also increased if over the years you have been calcium deficient, which you can discover by having a bone density test or by reviewing the calcium chart in appendix C. If part of your stomach or intestines were surgically removed, your body may not be absorbing enough calcium from the foods you eat. If you have chronic kidney disease, an overactive thyroid gland, or take thyroid drugs, or if you take bone-wasting drugs such as corticosteroids or heparin, the calcium balance in your body may be out of kilter.

The risk of osteoporosis may also be higher if you were deprived of female hormones before menopause or have never been pregnant, or if you have a family history of osteoporosis. The risks drop if you are muscular or overweight, or if you have taken estrogen after menopause for more than one year. They may also be lower if you used oral contraceptives for more than one year or were pregnant several times.

Some of these protective factors may seem surprising. Why overweight? Fatty tissue provides a compensatory mechanism against estrogen loss, so although being obese is definitely not a healthy option, being underweight is not desirable at midlife. Stringent dieting at this time can be detrimental. Physical exercise and muscularity may also protect you. If you are stronger and more agile because you exercise, you are less likely to fall and break bones. Exercise also improves your sense of well-being. In an elevated mood, you are less likely to take tranquilizers or sedatives that can lessen your coordination. That, too, can account for fewer falls and fewer fractures. Finally, weight-bearing exercise such as brisk walking may help to build and maintain bone density. The protective aspects of estrogen therapy, nutrition, and exercise together will be discussed in depth in chapters 5 through 8.

Measuring Bone Mass. Science has now made it possible to measure bone density. There are three good methods. The newest and best one is *dual x-ray absorptiometry,* which can accurately measure bone anywhere in the body. *Dual photon absorptiometry* also measures the amount of bone, but only in the spine or hip. *Computerized axial tomography* is a radiographic procedure, commonly referred to as a CAT scan, that can measure the spine accurately but uses higher x-ray doses and is more expensive.

We use these tests to measure the amount of bone tissue present in areas of the body that are fracture-prone like the spine and the hip joint. If the test is repeated twelve months later, we can accurately predict the likelihood of fractures in the future. This information enables us to recommend preventive care to women and to determine whether these measures are successful.

Cardiovascular System

We have only recently begun to consider heart disease as a women's issue. Yet cardiovascular disease is the number one killer of American women, claiming almost 400,000 lives each year. It was surprising to learn of the National Institutes of Health's finding that one in seven

SYMPTOMS CAUSED BY A DEFICIENCY OF
ESTROGEN/PROGESTERONE

Site	*Symptom/Problem*
PELVIC	
Vulva/vagina	Shrinkage, itching, painful intercourse, vaginal infection, blood-stained discharge
Uterus/pelvis	Prolapse (dropping of the uterus and the vagina)
Fallopian tubes	No symptoms
Bladder/urethra	Infection, change in the urethral opening, frequency and/or urgency of urination, inability to hold in urine
OTHER	
Neuroendocrine system	Hot flushes, sleep disorders such as insomnia or frequent waking
Breasts	Shrinking, sagging
Thyroid function	No known effect
Skeleton	Osteoporosis/related fractures, backache
Skin/mucous membranes	Atrophy, dryness, itching, easily bruised, loss of tone, dry hair or loss of hair, minor hairiness of the face, dry mouth
Cardiovascular	Atherosclerosis, angina, coronary heart disease

women, ages forty-five to sixty-four, has some form of heart disease, and that this number increases to one in three women over the age of sixty-five. It seems that heart disease does not limit itself to the ambitious hard-driving career-oriented woman or man. It can show up in anyone and may be related to the stresses of daily life, children, spouses, relatives, finances, and the demands of family life today.

The vastness of the problem of heart disease has led to a large number of research projects conducted over many years. We have learned that heredity plays a primary role and that certain forms of heart disease run in families. Beyond that, the most significant risk factors for heart disease rest with lifestyle choices that we can control. These include obesity, poor diet with high cholesterol and fat intake, cigarette smoking, lack of exercise, and stress. Other medical conditions such as hypertension (high blood pressure) and diabetes also increase our risk.

Research on coronary heart disease (CHD) in women has shown conclusively that there is a relationship between the function of the ovaries, the levels of hormones in the bloodstream, and the development of the plaque-like substances inside the blood vessels that eventually can cause blockage and lead to heart attacks. When medical science clarifies this relationship once and for all, it may be possible to understand the cause of heart disease in women in midlife and to prevent it.

Meanwhile, it is important to learn what you can do to reduce your risk of heart attack. Understanding the risk factors is a vital first step.

Heart Disease Risk Factors. Atherosclerosis is the form of heart disease for which all of the following risk factors are pertinent. It is a metabolic disease that is influenced by many factors and is the result of an accumulation of fatlike plaque on the arterial wall, a process that leads to the narrowing of the *coronary arteries* and can result in their blockage (coronary thrombosis). This blockage cuts off the blood supply to the heart and ultimately is responsible for a *heart attack* (myocardial infarction). *Arteriosclerosis* is a general term used to describe all cases in which these changes occur in the arteries.

Coronary risk factors can be broken down into those that affect all persons and those that are "women only" risk factors. Let's review them.

General Risk Factors

1. High blood cholesterol
2. Hypertension
3. Diabetes mellitus
4. Obesity
5. Poor diet
6. Cigarette smoking

7. Physical inactivity
8. Stress
9. Family history of heart disease

Women-Only Risk Factors

1. Menopause before age forty-five
2. Surgical menopause
3. Low estrogen level
4. Use of oral contraceptives

Early researchers found that, irrespective of age, women with functioning ovaries had less vascular disease than women who had already gone through menopause (either spontaneous or after surgical removal of the ovaries). These early clues led to investigations of larger populations. A study conducted in the town of Framingham, Massachusetts, where the entire adult population has been surveyed since 1949 for numerous risk factors for heart disease, confirmed these findings.

To understand fully the relationship between ovarian function and heart disease, investigators studied what happened to women who received some form of hormone replacement as compared to those who did not. In 1981, a study conducted of 20,000 residents of a Los Angeles retirement community by Ronald Ross, an epidemiologist, demonstrated that estrogen had a protective effect against CHD.

Of even more striking significance was that many studies, including a major study in Boston of 122,000 American nurses, showed that the risk of developing heart disease was increased in women who experienced menopause at a younger age. For example, women who experienced surgical menopause before the age of thirty-five carry two to seven times the risk of heart attack as premenopausal women with their ovaries intact.

The current medical opinion, based on this sound evidence, is that the ovary provides some protection against heart attacks, and that the younger a woman is when the ovary is removed or stops functioning, the greater her risk of heart attack. This increased risk can be negated if hormones are given as replacement therapy.

High blood cholesterol, cigarette smoking, and high blood pressure are important risk factors for coronary heart disease that lie outside of the sex-related differences outlined earlier.

Obesity. Obesity appears to be the most important risk factor for heart disease. The culprit in the diet is the type of fat that you eat, particularly the saturated fat that causes high *serum cholesterol.* Continuing studies of large groups of people have proved, beyond all reasonable doubt, that the risk of heart attack is directly related to the amount of fat (lipid) and cholesterol in the blood.

Cholesterol. High cholesterol, a waxy substance in the blood, can greatly increase your risk of developing CHD. If you have a high blood cholesterol level, you probably are getting too much cholesterol into your blood through the saturated fat and cholesterol in the foods that you eat. Genetic predisposition also plays a role in high cholesterol, but in most people cholesterol level is largely determined by diet. Besides, your body produces its own cholesterol, so if you ate none, it would still create enough for its needs.

Your risk for heart attack increases as your blood cholesterol rises. Information available in the United States shows that within the age range of thirty-five to forty-four years, the average cholesterol level is higher among men than women. However, a crossover occurs in the age range of forty-five to fifty-four, and after age fifty-five the average cholesterol levels for women are distinctly higher than those for men. This considerable increase in women's cholesterol levels as they age may be a response to the decrease in estrogen at menopause, but we are not sure.

Cholesterol, like wax, does not dissolve easily in water or in the blood. When plaque is found in the arteries, picture it as composed of fat, cholesterol, and collagen (the albuminlike protein in the body), sometimes along with deposits of calcium and cellular debris. If plaque builds up in an artery or blood vessel, it can clog it, closing it to the passage of blood. A heart attack occurs when this closure starves the heart for food and oxygen. A stroke occurs if plaque blocks the arteries to the brain. Obviously, a low cholesterol level in the blood is important so that the blood flows freely throughout your body.

Because cholesterol does not dissolve in blood, it must be carried in the blood by substances called *lipoproteins.* These, too, play a role in preventing heart disease. High-density lipoproteins (HDLs) are called the "good cholesterol." They remove excess cholesterol from the bloodstream and send it back to the liver for excretion. There are also two types of "bad cholesterol." These are the low-density lipoproteins (LDLs) and the very low-density lipoproteins (VLDLs).

LDLs carry cholesterol from the liver to the cells throughout the body after the VLDLs have carried their load of triglycerides from the liver to the tissues, where they form pockets of fat. Therefore, it is important to know your cholesterol level *and* your HDL and LDL levels.

More than half of all adult Americans have blood cholesterol levels greater than 200 mg/dl, which puts them at an increased risk for CHD. The National Cholesterol Education Program of the National Heart, Lung and Blood Institute at the National Institutes of Health has drawn up a classification for risk in relation to total cholesterol level.

National Institutes of Health's Guidelines on Total Cholesterol

less than 200 mg/dl	desirable blood cholesterol
200–239 mg/dl	borderline–high blood cholesterol
more than 240 mg/dl	high blood cholesterol

National Institutes of Health's Guidelines on LDL Cholesterol

less than 130 mg/dl	desirable LDL cholesterol
130–159 mg/dl	borderline–high-risk LDL cholesterol
more than 160 mg/dl	high-risk LDL cholesterol

To evaluate your serum cholesterol levels, your doctor will take a small amount of your blood. Your blood sample is sent to a laboratory and the test result is expressed as milligrams per deciliters, mg/dl. (This measurement refers to the amount of cholesterol found in a deciliter of liquid, which is the same as one-tenth of a liter or approximately one-tenth of a quart.) If your blood cholesterol level is found to be above 200 mg/dl, you should have the test repeated several times. Then use the average of those numbers to determine whether medical intervention is needed to lower your blood cholesterol. Any other CHD factors, such as high blood pressure, diabetes, obesity, smoking, family history, and personal medical history, should be taken into account if you have borderline high cholesterol. If you have your cholesterol tested at a public screening program, you should consult a physician if your level is found to be above 200 mg/dl.

Dietary treatment is the number one weapon in reducing cholesterol. It successfully lowers cholesterol for many people, reducing it to acceptable levels. Its main feature involves reducing your intake of saturated fat. Working with a qualified dietitian can help greatly if you are unsure about what to do. Obesity can also be the cause of high cholesterol levels. If you do have high cholesterol, it is helpful if you also have a high HDL level. Higher levels of the "good cholesterol" are found in people who exercise regularly, don't smoke, and who maintain a desirable weight.

These good health practices, all outlined in the Utian Program, can raise your HDL and help to offset, to some degree, a high total cholesterol level. If dietary changes do not reduce cholesterol levels sufficiently after six months, your physician may prescribe cholesterol-lowering drugs in conjunction with a low-cholesterol diet. Drug and diet therapy is advisable for individuals with an LDL cholesterol of 190 mg/dl or greater as well as for those with LDL cholesterol of 160–189 mg/dl who have CHD or two other risk factors. Lowering cholesterol has real benefit, slowing the fatty buildup in the arteries, and, in some cases, even reversing the process and reducing the risk of heart attack.

Cigarette Smoking. Cigarette smoking can cause CHD. Studies show that smoking narrows the blood vessels and slows the circulation of blood through the body, increasing the risk of vessel blockage and heart attack. Smoking is also the major single cause of cancer, accounting for some 30 percent of such deaths in the United States annually.

The 1986 Report of the Surgeon General, *The Health Consequences of Involuntary Smoking,* extends the health risks of tobacco smoke to the nonsmoker as well: Passive smoking can cause disease in healthy nonsmokers. The children of smokers have more frequent respiratory infections, more respiratory problems, and slightly inferior lung function as compared to children of nonsmokers. Sadly, separating smokers from nonsmokers in a common space does not eliminate the risk to nonsmokers, although it may reduce the risk slightly.

In women, we know that smoking speeds up the onset of menopause. This fact may explain in part the increased rate of heart attack in women who smoke. We also know that women who smoke are thinner than nonsmokers and that leaness is also associated with a slightly earlier menopause.

Blood Pressure. Young women have lower blood pressure than young men, but this difference also decreases with age. In the Framingham study, blood pressure was found to be distinctly higher in midlife women and was associated with a higher incidence of heart attacks.

Q. **How can I protect myself against CHD?**

A. Younger women are less vulnerable than men to heart attacks, but their relative protection decreases as they become older. Now that we understand how estrogen deficiency in menopause may be a major coronary risk factor for women, we caution you to hold onto your ovaries, if possible, when undergoing hysterectomy. There are other significant risk factors that you can control, such as avoiding obesity by reducing fats in your diet, and stopping smoking. You can't change your heredity, but you can minimize all the other factors that are within your power to control.

Q. **Are women genetically programmed to age differently from one another?**

A. Of course, women do not look alike and are not built the same, but what may be startling news is that women may vary even *more* after menopause. These differences were first noted in studies conducted in Scandinavia in the early 1960s. The subjects of the study were women who were about to undergo hysterectomies that included removal of both ovaries. Before surgery, complete medical histories were taken and the amount of sex hormones in the women's bodies was measured. Following surgery, the same hormones were measured again and the medical history was repeated. The ovaries, removed during surgery, were analyzed and a technique called *histochemical staining* was performed to learn whether they were producing hormones.

The remarkable findings of these investigations are that there were stunning differences in postmenopausal women that separated them into two distinct groups. The more youthful-appearing group of women who had fewer symptoms before surgery had elevated levels of sex hormones, particularly two called *androstenedione*, a weak male hormone, and *estrone,* one of the three female estrogens. These hormone levels declined after surgery, when the women began to experience postmenopausal symptoms—in particular, hot flashes. Further, the removed ovaries from this group indicated that, when intact, they had been producing sex hormones. In contrast, the older-appearing group of women had the same low levels of sex hormone production before and after surgery. Their removed ovaries were atrophied, scarred, and had been incapable of producing sex hormones.

What do these findings mean? They mean that some women have inherent compensatory mechanisms that guard against some of the precipitous hormone changes and problems that can occur after menopause. These mechanisms include differences in the structure of the postmenopausal ovaries, variations in the amounts of male hormone they have that can be converted to female hormone, and differences in the way their hormones are transported in their bodies.

These compensatory mechanisms may explain why some women are not as uncomfortable during menopause as others. They may also explain why there are variations among women in their need for or response to hormone replacement therapy (HRT).

Q. Why are ovaries removed?
A. The ovaries are sometimes removed with the uterus in a surgical procedure called *hysterectomy*. Taking out normal ovaries during a routine hysterectomy is medically controversial. It is a subject that each woman facing hysterectomy should discuss thoroughly with her own physician. The reasons often cited for removing healthy ovaries at the time of hysterectomy include the following:

- To prevent later development of ovarian cancer—a very slim risk set at somewhere between 1 in 1,000 to 1 in 3,000 hysterectomies and often offset by the ovaries' protective value in preventing heart disease and osteoporosis.
- To forestall the risk that ovaries, when left behind, might cease to work properly—a theory that is simply not true for most women.
- To prevent future surgery to remove ovarian cysts—which may never develop.

Well-founded reasons for the removal of the ovaries during surgery include taking out ovaries that no longer function because the woman is past menopause, or if she is premenopausal but over the age of fifty because the ovary has a short future. If a woman wants her ovaries removed during hysterectomy, that is her prerogative, once she has been fully informed of the consequences. If the hysterectomy is being done because of pelvic cancer, in which case the ovaries would be destroyed by radiation therapy anyway, or if it is surgically impossible to save them because of the woman's history of pelvic infection, or if the ovaries are in any other way diseased, then the ovaries must be removed. There are far more compelling reasons for leaving healthy ovaries intact:

- To prevent the menopausal symptoms that follow their removal.
- To prevent changes in other body organs, such as skin, breasts, and vagina that occur due to the loss of ovarian hormones.
- To prevent osteoporosis.
- To prevent earlier onset of the risk of heart attack.
- To prevent unnecessary psychological and physical stress.

Q. Can menopause occur early?

A. Premature, or early, menopause can be caused in many ways. The number one culprit is the surgical removal of the ovaries in premenopausal women. Even when there are valid reasons for removing them, the postmenopausal problems that follow are usually more severe than in natural menopause because of the suddenness of the ovarian removal.

Other factors that may influence the early onset of menopause include cigarette smoking. The Boston Collaborative Drug Surveillance Program analysis of two large independent sets of data showed that heavy smokers were more likely to go through menopause earlier. If you have smoked and stopped, your chances of early menopause are increased compared to women who have never smoked, but early menopause is less likely when compared to a current smoker. Why this is true is yet unexplained, but two theories exist. One is that the contents of cigarette smoke cause the liver to destroy estrogen. The other suggests that nicotine reduces the blood supply to the ovary, which, lacking nourishment, may shrivel.

Beyond this information, we do not know why the ovary fails prematurely. It has been theorized that it may happen because for some reason the body develops antibodies that attack ovarian tissue or block the function of the follicle stimulating hormone (FSH) described earlier. Further research is underway to learn what really causes premature natural menopause.

Q. So what should I expect during the climacteric?

A. I advise my patients to consider the climacteric as one syndrome that occurs over a period of time. If you understand it as such, it is easier to see that not all the symptoms of menopause will affect all women at the same point in their climacteric. Thus, the whole experience, while shared by all women, can be very different for each woman. The following chart may help explain this concept.

This chart graphically explains the range of individual differences in women's climacteric experiences, showing that the tissues change at different rates in women. Some women will be more affected than others by these changes. Physicians, however, must be equally concerned about the woman who has no apparent discomfort from menopause, since she may be quickly and quietly losing bone in such quantity that she may be a candidate for osteoporosis.

THE STAGES AND SYMPTOMS
OF THE CLIMACTERIC CONTINUUM

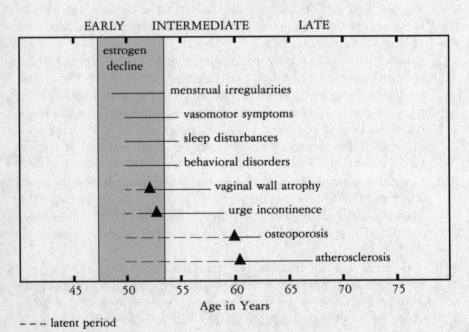

--- latent period

▲——— symptom manifest

Source: Adapted from Utian, W. H.: *Menopause in Modern Perspective,* 1980.

The longer the negative effects of menopause are allowed to continue, the more likely it is that problems can develop. To see where you are in the intricate process of menopause, fill out the menopause questionnaire at the end of chapter 4.

Many women are not aware that there may be a long period of transition into the climacteric that starts many years before menopause is even considered. I call this period the "PMS of menopause," or *premenopausal syndrome,* which is described in the next chapter.

·4·

*Your Helpful
Early Warning System*

Does PMS Also Mean *Premenopausal* Syndrome?

Once a month Queen Victoria would become unaccountably en-
raged at Prince Albert, screaming accusations and hurling any
object that came to hand across the room. If the royal consort tried
to reason with her, she would shriek more loudly and vitupera-
tively. If he remained silent, he would be accused of insulting the
royal presence. If he withdrew to his room, Victoria would pound
on his door with her tiny fists . . . the Queen suffered from a classic
case of premenstrual syndrome.

> Matt Clark and Dan Shapiro
> *Newsweek,* May 14, 1981

Assiduously kept menstrual charts showed that three young female
convicts imprisoned for repeated criminal acts ranging from theft
to murder *only* broke the law during their premenstrual days.

> K. Dalton, *Lancet* 2:1070, 1981

Premenstrual syndrome (PMS) may be the newest women's health
issue in the United States. Some severely affected women are now
going public with their stories and are demanding treatment.

> Editorial, *Journal of the
> American Medical Association* 245:1393, 1981

In the early 1980s, the "monthly difficulties" of many women and
their profound effects on family, career, and society became national
news. Could it be that many women who were plagued by mood
swings and physical discomfort for several days each month were

experiencing something *real* about which they lacked information and over which they had no control?

Was PMS real? The public began to think so. The long-awaited recognition of PMS by the medical and the media communities empowered women in their own behalf. They could, at last, quit apologizing for their actions and start taking action instead. Let's look at what happened to one of my patients. I'll call her Claire.

The Story of Claire

"There is no way to describe how awful PMS is for me and for my husband and my children. They can't possibly understand what I go through each month or why my relationship with them resembles an emotional rollercoaster ride."

I recalled Claire's statement vividly and actually wrote it in her chart because it demonstrates the complicated and far-reaching effects of premenstrual syndrome (PMS) in a poignant way that I always want to remember. Claire is thirty-four years old and the mother of two daughters: one age nine and the other age seven. She came to see me because she felt that her life was suddenly collapsing.

Claire described her daily activities. The problems of her busy daily schedule consumed her and yet she was lonely. She perceived herself to be living a life apart from her loving, ambitious, workaholic husband. Their daughters' school activities seemed to lurch from catastrophe to catastrophe, which Claire felt compelled to handle alone since her husband's work kept him so busy. It didn't help that their dog was about to give birth to its third litter of puppies momentarily, a fact that seemed overwhelming to Claire. She expressed embarrassment at discussing these matters with me, because she had always prided herself on being in complete control of herself and her life. But in the past eighteen months she told me that nothing seemed to be going right.

Always a clear thinker, Claire was alarmed when she began to experience episodes of forgetfulness and helplessness. She had frequent headaches. Worst of all, she was totally unable to control her emotions. She screamed at the girls for the slightest reason, and at her husband for even less. She reported that he initially responded quietly, but that eventually he began to fight back. Something deep down inside her signaled that these tumultuous battles had to end. However, she could not stop becoming upset about almost everything.

Then one evening in the middle of an argument, her husband called her "crazy" and said she was in need of psychiatric care. Claire knew, then, that it was time to seek help. Coincidentally, she received her card from our office reminding her that it was time for her annual Pap test. During her visit to my office, she told me her story and asked for help. We talked throughout her physical examination, the results of which were normal.

Then we sat in my office and talked further. Claire spoke of her "chaotic life." She was unable to pinpoint her "anger attacks," but agreed that they might be cyclical, although until now she had not suffered any symptoms of premenstrual discomfort. She did not remember her mother or her two older sisters having this problem. She did know that her mother had become menopausal at the age of forty-three and that her sisters had entered menopause in their mid-forties.

My first treatment tactic was to reassure Claire that she was not going "crazy." The next was to ask her to start a monthlong "mood and symptom inventory," by carefully charting her feelings and physical symptoms throughout an entire menstrual cycle. At our next appointment, we reviewed the mood chart. It confirmed that her "bad days" occurred in the last ten days before the onset of her period.

There are no confirming tests for PMS: Not even a blood test will clinch the diagnosis. So we had to depend on Claire's detailed medical history, the fact that her medical examination showed that she had no other organic disease, the additional fact of her mother's and sisters' early menopause, the entries on her symptom chart, and her diet survey, which indicated she regularly consumed a lot of coffee, cheese, and chocolate. These are all foods that can make PMS worse.

Now the work began. Claire needed to eliminate coffee, cheese, and chocolate from her diet, begin to exercise regularly, and take progesterone in the second half of her cycle. (Although unproven scientifically at this time, progesterone therapy does help some women who are suffering from PMS.) This treatment program led to a quick response and soon she experienced complete relief of her symptoms.

There is little doubt in my mind that Claire's problem was caused by her unusually severe reaction to the subtle hormonal changes that were taking place in her body in the decade before menopause. The fact that we were able to help her illustrates that there are simple methods that can bring great relief from PMS, a condition that can be a life-shattering experience for some women.

New Insights About PMS

Once upon a time, not very long ago, a woman who approached her physician with the complaint of problems related to her menstrual cycle was blithely told that "it was all in her mind." Perhaps, in some ways, that diagnosis was right, although it was pronounced for the wrong reasons. The symptoms that some women describe *are* probably in the mind, but as a result of chemical interactions and imbalances in the brain, not because of some psychological disorder.

We know that the increase in estrogen during a woman's normal reproductive cycle is associated with mood enhancement and that the decrease in hormones around the onset of menstruation can create a downswing in mood. When the degree of mood change is severe, the problem is now usually called premenstrual syndrome or premenstrual tension.

The most recent medical findings make it clear that premenstrual syndrome is not a simple hormone deficiency or imbalance. Rather, it appears that the brain's reaction to normal hormone levels will vary under different circumstances. One of these circumstances may be the process of reproductive aging itself.

We now know that there is a group of premenstrual syndromes and that individual women react differently to them with body, mind, perception, and behavior disturbances. We call one of these premenstrual syndromes *premenopausal syndrome.* Premenopausal syndrome appears to be a specific early indicator of impending menopause.

Does the M in PMS Stand for Menopause?

If you read any book or article about PMS, you will notice that it is invariably accompanied by a long list of symptoms. In our opinion, creating such a list is futile and could even be counterproductive, because the syndrome is so variable. Some of the symptoms can occur in relation to your monthly cycle, and many of the symptoms can— once having occurred—also change during your cycle. The same symptom can affect other women in very different ways. There is no group of symptoms that uniformly and regularly affects each individual woman.

If you think you might have PMS, the best way to determine how the syndrome affects you is to chart any changes in perception, behavior, and feeling that you experience during your monthly cycle using the format described earlier for Claire. Physical symptoms could include breast tenderness and swelling, abdominal bloating, edema, and weight gain. Emotional symptoms often include anxiety, depression, tension, insomnia, anger, and fear. Behavioral changes sometimes have included absenteeism from work, proneness to accidents, and in very rare instances, other phenomena such as criminal tendencies and suicidal impulses.

The variety of symptoms of PMS can make diagnosis difficult. The best way to begin involves giving your physician a very detailed history. You will also probably be asked to chart your symptoms carefully, measure your body weight on a daily basis, and record your entire behavioral pattern over two to three monthly menstrual cycles. Your doctor, then, has a basis for evaluation. (A PMS diagnostic chart has been included to help you chart your symptoms. Take the chart to your physician.)

Since many theories relate PMS to hormonal changes, you may wonder why physicians do not simply measure the amount of estrogen and progesterone in your blood. Unfortunately, this practice does not offer the easy answer it seems to suggest. Your hormonal changes may be so subtle that your hormone measurements fall within accepted normal limits even though your body is reacting strongly to those changes. So these blood tests will merely be expensive for you and will not help to diagnose your problem.

Studies of hormonal levels in premenstrual syndrome have shown a striking lack of consistency. For example, comparisons of hormone levels in both women with and without PMS have failed to show any statistical differences between the two groups. This lack of difference shows that PMS is not caused by abnormal circulating levels of gonadotropins or gonadal hormones.

Other hormones such as prolactin, cortisol, and thyroid hormone have been thought to be possible causes of PMS. However, no substantiated medical reports exist as yet to confirm this theory. Other investigators have tried to relate symptoms such as irritability, aggression, and paranoia to higher levels of male hormone within the female body. Studies have also failed to confirm this relationship.

PMS DIAGNOSTIC CHART
Utian Menopause Management Program

Instructions: Chart from first day of period (bleeding) until the first day of the next cycle. Enter a check mark for each day of bleeding. Enter date of onset of period. Every night, check *one box only* under the appropriate cycle day number for Items #1 through #4. Circle appropriate symptoms in Item #5.

Important: This is a simplified PMS chart designed only to give introductory information to your physician. It is not a complete PMS diagnostic system.

Date Period Started: _____

Day of Cycle:	1	2	3	4	5	6	7	8	9	10	11	12	13	14	15	16	17	18	19	20	21	22	23	24	25	26	27	28	29	30	31	32	33	34	35	36	37	38	39	40
Bleeding (✓)																																								
1. *My Mood Today Is*																																								
Lousy																																								
Wonderful																																								
Normal																																								
2. *My Body Felt*																																								
Bloated																																								
Uncomfortable																																								
Normal																																								
3. *My Life Was*																																								
Not Affected																																								
Sad																																								
Happy																																								
Miserable																																								
4. *Outside Events Were*																																								
Great																																								
Bad																																								
Non-Specific																																								

5. *Circle your most troublesome symptoms:*

Depressed   Irritable   Tired   Angry   Breast Pain   Headache   Weight Gain   Anxious   Insomnia   Menstrual Cramps   Edema

55

Since it seems that we cannot blame PMS on hormone imbalances, we are led to theorize that PMS may be the result of abnormal responses to normal endocrine levels. Research today is directed toward more sophisticated evaluations to learn what actually occurs chemically in the brain.

When large groups of women with premenstrual symptoms were studied, the results suggested that PMS actually may be clusters of problems that can occur separately at different phases in a woman's life. One of these phases is the premenopausal time. It is likely that women who have few PMS symptoms in their early reproductive years, but who suddenly develop such symptoms in their later reproductive years, may be suffering from a variant of PMS that should appropriately be called *premenopausal syndrome.*

Treating PMS

Because doctors do not know the definitive cause of premenstrual tension, there are as many different kinds of treatments offered to women as there are symptoms. Some doctors proclaim hormone treatment successful, but research studies do not support this claim. Nonetheless, many women request—and many physicians continue to prescribe—hormone treatment. Until something better comes along, if it seems to work, hormone treatment is certainly worth trying. In the United Kingdom, Dr. Katherina Dalton reported success with natural progesterone, which has become one of the most popular of the hormone therapies.

Other hormone therapies that sometimes have brought relief include estrogen, combinations of estrogen and progestin (the subject of current medical debate) and, more recently, estrogen implants. Physicians have also tried to help PMS sufferers by suggesting that they take vitamins and minerals and eliminate food additives, but the success with these routes of treatment has not been dramatic. Not one treatment has proved to be more satisfactory than any other. Unfortunately, I cannot show you a clear path leading to total relief from PMS. Yet, I hope that it is reassuring to know that if you have symptoms of this nature, there is a medical reason for your distress, even though a cause has not been pinpointed and the medical treatments discovered so far may not have helped you.

If you suffer from PMS, besides a careful program of medication, healthy diet, and regular exercise, you may value the emotional support of group sessions that offer relaxation techniques to ease depression. One of the best roads to successful therapy is to find a physician who understands PMS, is sympathetic to your problem, and who may be able to suggest a support group that will offer substantial emotional support.

Other Early Warning Signs of Menopause

Even though late-arriving PMS can be an early symptom of menopause, there are four other physical symptoms that can occur that are even stronger indicators of early menopause. We include them here so that you can be aware of them, but do not worry about them. They are all easily treated, if treatment is required.

Hot Flushes or Flashes

There is still a strange resistance among physicians to accept the fact that hot flashes can occur long before the end of menstruation—as early as age thirty-five. The symptom may cause you to feel warmth spreading across your face and throughout your body. It may be followed by perspiration, and then you may feel cold, or even begin to shiver. The hot flash can be so severe that you become drenched with sweat and feel emotionally drained. When it occurs at night it may awaken you from sleep and is accurately called a "night sweat." Hot flashes can occur at irregular intervals, and, occasionally, with extreme frequency. They also vary in severity, from being a slight nuisance to causing a major disruption in the quality of your life. You might never connect these early flashes to menopause, because your menstrual periods will continue, but if you experience these symptoms, be aware that your body is beginning its midlife transition on the early side. Be sure to alert your physician to that fact and follow the hot flash relief guidelines later in this chapter.

Abnormal Periods

Another early warning sign may be an unexplained change in the nature of your menstrual flow or menstrual pattern. You may notice that the amount of bleeding lessens each month and, eventually, stops entirely. It is a comfortable way for menopause to start. Sometimes the periods stop abruptly, which gives you no advance warning of menopause approaching. Other less convenient changes can occur in your menstrual period. For example, it can last for seven days one month and only three the next, or you may go for an unusually long stretch of time without periods. As a result, you never quite know where you are in your cycle, and your period can take you by surprise. Sometimes your period may not only be irregular in onset and duration but the amount of bleeding may vary: heavy one month; light the next. In some instances, the bleeding can be so heavy that you feel weak, dizzy, or otherwise concerned, and you may need to see your physician.

Bladder Control
You may notice that as menopause approaches you seem to have less control over your bladder. This problem may start as a little leaking of urine during moments of muscular stress, such as during exercise, running, or jogging, or simply when laughing or sneezing. It is a common occurrence when estrogen levels in your system begin to drop, which may cause a slackening of your muscular pelvic floor and of the control mechanism of the bladder as well.

Changes in Short-Term Memory
Recently, decreasing estrogen levels were linked to changes in short-term memory. The ability to remember immediate events, like the items on your shopping list, or to recall where you left your car keys or sunglasses can be attributed to declining estrogen levels. Unfortunately, not all lapses of memory can be blamed on this common symptom, but if you are experiencing short-term memory loss more often, don't panic. Consider that it might be a warning that menopause is approaching.

What Younger Women Should Know about Getting Older

Getting older is terrific and very natural! It's what we all begin to do at the moment of our birth. If you could just keep that same happy anticipation that you felt while waiting to "become a woman" for your final menstrual period, you could quite contentedly look forward to what's in store for you in the future.

Maybe the nomenclature is deceiving. The word *climacteric* comes from the Greek and means "critical time." Sometime during this so-called critical time, (generally a ten-year span between the ages of forty-five and fifty-five) your last period will occur—usually when you're around the age of fifty. But changes are happening long before that time, and beginning in your thirties, you may not only notice them but you can do something about them. Best of all, you can thwart any harmful results of these changes when you observe and catch them early.

The number of eggs that your ovaries produce will lessen and stop sometime during the climacteric. You cannot see or feel or reverse those universal changes. However, you can alleviate many of the other bodily changes that occur as a result of the cessation of menses. The hot flash is the most prevalent sign and can start early. Almost all women have them at menopause. The hot flash can make you feel as if your personal thermostat has gone awry. Suddenly, you are uncomfortably hot. While you are removing your jacket or sweater, you realize that no one else in the room is feeling the heat. So it begins. For many women, the hot flash is just a mild discomfort, yet others sweat through intense heat. For some, the hot flash occurs only occasionally; for others it returns with almost unbearable regularity.

You may be able to avoid hot flashes or lessen their intensity by avoiding alcohol, especially red wine (the chemicals in it seem to encourage flashes and headaches), and tobacco, caffeine, and stress (whenever possible). Regular exercise helps, too, to stabilize your body. Relaxation and visualization techniques, in which you conjure up cool, comfortable surroundings, may work for you as well.

If you are in your mid-thirties and beginning to show premenopausal symptoms, you can begin to work toward having a more comfortable menopause by following the diet outlined in chapter 7 and by exercising regularly to protect yourself against heart disease and to conserve bone mass to help safeguard you against osteoporosis. Exercise is so important that we devoted all of chapter 8 to it, but we should mention here also that the activities that help the younger women most are weight-bearing pursuits such as racquet sports, walking, cross-country skiing, low-impact aerobic dancing, and bicycling.

Vaginal discomfort can occur early, too, as the vaginal lining gradually thins in response to very subtle shifts in estrogen levels. Some women in their thirties do experience vaginal dryness, itching, and atrophy, causing some discomfort during sexual activity. Frequent sex is the most positive prescription for these problems. If you are at a time in your life when it takes you longer to become sexually aroused and lubricated, then tell your caring partner openly. If extra lubrication is necessary, consider using a vaginal moisturizer like Replens. If more than that seems required, check with your physician to see if a vaginal estrogen cream should be prescribed for you.

Bladder control problems can occur with estrogen decline because the muscles in the pelvic area become slacker or weaker. Certain exercises can help to keep that muscle strong. Kegel exercises, named for the physician who first described them, usually work. There are two varieties: the slow Kegel, during which you contract all the pelvic muscles as if you were trying to squeeze the vaginal opening closed, holding it closed for a count of three, relaxing, and doing it again; and the fast Kegel, in which you alternately contract and relax the muscle as quickly as you can. Twelve of these exercises each time you stop at a traffic signal for a total of fifty Kegels per day will often work wonders with bladder control and may enhance your sex life, too.

We know that aging is more difficult in a youth-oriented society such as ours, and far easier to accept in other cultures where age and wisdom are synonymous and revered. However, change is change, and for some people it is always exciting; for others it is always stressful. Our ability to handle change has to do with matching positive actions to a positive attitude about the change. Thus, the Utian Menopause Management Program can be a valuable asset to your continued good health. It promotes a positive outlook and shows you how to structure your diet, exercise program, health and grooming practices, and vocations, avocations, and preventive medicine programs to get the best out of the best years, which are yet to come.

As you enter midlife, many changes occur that you should know about in order to find the health maintenance program that is best for you. PMS, when it arrives late in your reproductive life, may be a premenopausal signal that it is time to spend some time on yourself. The following questionnaire was designed to help you figure out just where you fit into the midlife cycle. Once you know, you can make optimal use of the Utian Menopause Management Program. Your responses may also serve as a foundation for your next meeting with your physician.

The Menopause Questionnaire

1. How old were you when you had your first period? _____
2. Have your periods stopped? _____

3. Are you missing periods? _____

4. Is your cycle very irregular? _____

5. What was the date of your last period? _____

6. How old were you when you had your final period? _____
   If your periods have stopped, answer questions 7 to 10.

7. Did you suffer pain with your periods? Yes____No____

8. Did you suffer with premenstrual symptoms? Yes____No____

9. If so, what were your worst symptoms? _____
   _____
   _____

10. Have you experienced bleeding following menopause?
    Yes____No____

    If premenopausal, answer questions 11 to 16.

11. To check for PMS, read through this list and indicate any symp-
    toms that you often experience in the week before your period.

Tender breasts	Yes____	No____
Swollen breasts	Yes____	No____
Abdominal fullness	Yes____	No____
Abdominal pain	Yes____	No____
Tiredness	Yes____	No____
Sadness	Yes____	No____
Confusion	Yes____	No____
Pessimism	Yes____	No____
Weight gain	Yes____	No____
Tenseness	Yes____	No____
Nausea	Yes____	No____
Headaches	Yes____	No____
Irritability	Yes____	No____
Slow performance	Yes____	No____

12. Approximately how many days are there now from the first day
    of one period to the first day of your next period? _____days.
    If this has been varying a lot lately, describe how. _____
    _____
    _____

13. Approximately how many days does your period usually last
    now? _____days. If this has been changing a lot lately,
    describe how.

The following questions will help to determine whether you are in the perimenopausal period.

Compared with five years ago,
14. I get my periods: More often ( )   Less often ( )
15. My periods last: Longer ( )   Shorter ( )
16. The bleeding is: Heavier ( )   Lighter ( )

Think about your family history.

17. Do you have a family history of any of the following?
Osteoporosis_____ Stroke_____ Coronary thrombosis_____
Breast cancer_____ Diabetes_____ Uterine cancer_____
Hypertension_____ Others_____

Think about your surgical history. Have you had any of these operations? If so, how old were you?

18. Tubes tied   Yes_____ No_____ Age_____
19. Vaginal repair   Yes_____ No_____ Age_____
20. Hysterectomy   Yes_____ No_____ Age_____
21. Ovaries removed   Yes_____ No_____ Age_____
    If yes: Right_____Left_____Both_____
22. If you had a hysterectomy, why was it done? _____
_____
_____

23. Were you depressed or did you experience any other psychological problem after your hysterectomy?
    Yes ( )____Severely____Moderately____Mildly____No ( )____
24. How long did the symptoms last? _____
25. Do you still have them?   Yes ( ) No ( )

Let's review your gynecological history.

26. Have you ever taken contraceptive pills? _____
27. Do you still take them? _____
28. How long have you taken them? _____
29. Have you ever used the intrauterine device (IUD)? _____
30. Do you have any vaginal discharge other than blood at any time?_____

31. Do you have an itch or irritation in the vagina? _____
32. Do you bleed after sexual intercourse? _____

Let's see whether you are postmenopausal.

33. Is your vagina dry during intercourse? _____
34. Is your vagina sore during intercourse? _____
35. Is your vagina dry or uncomfortable at other times? _____
36. Do you ever feel a "dropping" feeling in your vagina? _____
37. Do you get hot flushes? _____
38. How much do flushes bother you?
    Not at all____ Slightly____ Moderately____ A lot____
    Extremely____
39. Below is a list of some of the ways in which hot flushes can concern women. Please indicate how you feel about your hot flashes.
    Embarrassed ( ) Irritated ( ) Agitated (jittery) ( ) Uncomfortable ( ) Frightened ( ) Tense ( ) Sweaty ( ) Tired/weak ( ) Hot ( ) Faint ( )
    Any others? _____
40. About how many times a day do you have flushes? _____
41. How many times do you have them at night? _____
42. Do they interfere with: Work?_____ Sleep? _____
43. When did they begin: Before your periods stopped? _____ When your periods stopped?_____A while after your periods stopped?_____
44. How long have you had flushes? _____
45. Do you know of anything that makes them more likely to occur? If so, describe. _____
46. Have you had estrogen therapy for menopausal problems?____ If so, for how long?_____When? _____
47. If you stopped hormone replacement therapy, when did you stop? _____
48. Do you need to pass urine more often? _____
49. Do you lose urine under stress? _____
50. Do you ever hurt or burn when you urinate? _____
51. Did you begin to have headaches after menopause? _____

Now let's see if you are helping yourself at midlife.

52. Do you smoke?_____Drink alcohol regularly?_____Follow a diet?_____Eat dairy products often?_____Take calcium?_____Drink more than five cups of coffee per day? _____Eat red meat more than four times a week?_____ Drink soda more than once a day?_____

53. In general, do you feel better or worse since menopause began? Better_____Same_____Worse_____

54. Do you have sexual intercourse as frequently as you would like?
_____

55. Did you have sexual intercourse more often five years ago? ___

56. How have your feelings about sexual intercourse changed? Desire_____Enjoyment_____ Physical discomfort_____Dry vagina_____Sore vagina_____ Orgasm_____

57. What kind of exercise do you do? _____ How often?_____For how long? _____

58. Do you believe that you can improve the quality of your life through planned preventive programs? _____

59. Do you generally feel happy about this time in your life? _____

60. Are you ready to begin the Utian Menopause Management Program?

We hope that filling out this questionnaire has been an illuminating experience for you. It should have underscored those lifestyle choices that you have made that are good for you and indicated those where you might consider change. It also may be useful in communicating with your own physician about your individual midlife concerns.

It should be clear by now that menopause is merely a marker in the chronology of your life. We believe that women's lives should be viewed on a continuum and that the late reproductive years, from age thirty-five to menopause, should be considered the early climacteric. During this phase, the system of early-warning signals outlined in this chapter may let you know of impending changes. These are nature's helpful signs that indicate that this is a good time to begin a preventive healthcare program, such as the Utian Menopause Management Program, to assure a healthy and happy trip through the second half of life.

·5·

Taking Control of Your Life

What Hormone Replacement Therapy and Other Tools Can Do for You

Most of the changes that happen to your body when your hormone production slows down can be prevented, and many others can be reversed. This chapter describes the kinds of treatments that are available for preventive or protective therapy.

Exciting scientific advances in the last fifty years have given rise to whole new groups of hormonal and nonhormonal medications for use during and after menopause. These are not remedies prescribed over the telephone or obtained over the counter, but ones that must be discussed with and carefully prescribed by your own physician and taken under your doctor's supervision.

There is nothing new about the theory of "rejuvenation" therapy. Ancient Egyptians introduced organotherapy, or glandular therapy, and ate the penis of the ass for this purpose. Ancient Greeks and Romans changed the prescription to asses' testicles. Early scientists of the 1800s added other ideas to that kind of treatment. More than one hundred years ago, in 1888, a seventy-two-year-old famous French physiologist, Brown-Sequard, reported that he had rejuvenated himself by taking injections of "testicular juice." He wrote that he achieved greater body vigor, improved bladder and intestinal function, and that his wife used the testicular extract to combat feminine discomforts.

By the close of the nineteenth century, ovarian therapy started, with ovarian juice, powdered ovaries, and powdered ovarian tablets prescribed for surgical menopause, dysmenorrhea, and obesity. In 1926,

A. S. Parkes and C. W. Bellerby, two scientists in Great Britain, extracted female hormone from an ovary for the first time. They named it *estrin.* A few years later, a German chemist, A. Butenandt, isolated and synthesized a pure form of estrogen and progesterone. He won the Nobel Prize for his work. Now that these hormones were available, physicians prescribed them for a wide range of women's symptoms.

The wholesale prescription of this treatment became so popular that by the 1960s many books and articles ascribed all sorts of value to it, but did not describe any of the risks. The use of these powerful hormones escalated. Physicians and women alike were shocked when, in December 1975, scientific papers were released showing a causal relationship between hormone therapy and cancer of the uterus.

Women became afraid to use these medications. Fear, coupled with confusion and combined with a lack of comprehensive information, reigned. The only redeeming feature of this frightening dilemma was that scientists, physicians, and paramedical specialists finally began to conduct intensive research on the phenomenon of menopause. As a result, today physicians are able to reassure women because they have a fuller understanding of how menopause works. They now know much more about how the hormones function, how they can safely be prescribed, and what other forms of observation and treatment are necessary for their female patients.

While hormone replacement therapy (HRT) for postmenopausal women continues to be somewhat controversial, it is growing in popularity. Earlier, we described how the ovary starts to lose certain hormones and what happens to women as a result. Remember, too, that this hormone deficiency is more severe in some women than in others. The purpose of HRT is to make up for that deficiency. Not all women can take HRT, and not all women need to, as we'll explain more fully later in this chapter and in chapter 6. For women who can, and who choose to, HRT holds the promise of preventing or reversing many of the negative effects on the body caused by the lack of estrogen.

Good Reasons for Taking HRT

There are several compelling reasons for taking HRT. Carefully prescribed and safely taken, HRT offers the following:

- Relief from hot flushes, flashes, and related vasomotor symptoms
- Relief of vaginal atrophy and other pelvic atrophic conditions
- Maintenance of skin: keeping it smoother, thicker, and softer
- Prevention of osteoporosis and reduction of risk of fractures
- Protection against coronary heart disease and heart attack
- Benefits to the central nervous system including improvement of memory and of sleep, and the general enhancement of well-being and sexuality

The factors listed above can make a big difference in the quality and the quantity of your life, if you are, or when you become, postmenopausal. If HRT is so good, you may wonder why doctors don't give hormones to every woman. Some women do not need HRT and others cannot take it.

Who Is Eligible for Hormone Replacement Therapy?

HRT cannot be provided for some women because of other preexisting conditions or illnesses, or because they do not need it. If your well-informed doctor does not recommend hormones for you after you both discuss them as an option, he or she is most likely making this decision with your best interests in mind. In practice, I do not prescribe HRT if a woman has any of the following:

- Known or suspected breast or uterine cancer or any other estrogen-dependent tumor (a tumor in which estrogen will stimulate growth)
- Strong family history of estrogen-dependent cancers
- Abnormal and unexplained genital bleeding
- Dubin-Johnson syndrome (chronic jaundice—a liver problem) or chronic liver disease
- Acute liver disease

There are other conditions that are not conclusive reasons for withholding HRT, but call for an especially careful evaluation before estrogen can be prescribed. In most of these situations, some form of adequate hormone replacement can be worked out.

- Uterine fibroids
- Endometriosis
- Hyperlipidemia or hypercholesterolemia (conditions of abnormally high concentrations of fat or cholesterol in the blood)
- Severe varicose veins
- Diabetes mellitus
- Porphyria (metabolic disturbance that can cause acute abdominal or nervous problem, or photosensitivity of the skin or sores on its surface)
- Severe hypertension
- Previous or present thromboembolism, or severe thrombophlebitis

A combination of risk factors, such as obesity and liver disease, could also be a reason not to take HRT. Thus, it is important for you and your doctor to work out the ratio of benefit to risk before making a decision about HRT for you.

Different Kinds of HRT

The only hormones we will discuss here are the female sex hormones in the estrogen and progesterone categories. (There is a male hormone, testosterone, which we don't use very often in the treatment of women any longer, but it is listed in appendix A for your information.) The names estrogen and progesterone signify two groups of hormones. Each can be subclassified. Each of these subtypes has chemical names that we call *generic* names. These generically named drugs can be packaged or bottled separately or in mixtures, or may even be included with other drugs. The resulting commercial package ends up in your drugstore with a different name, which is its *trade* name.

Internationally, physicians accept the generic names: The trade names often differ from country to country. Moreover, some drugs are available in some countries, whereas others are not. It depends on the local regulations and the dictates of authorities such as the Food and Drug Administration (FDA) in the United States.

Until the early 1950s, there were no progesterone medications that were helpful when taken orally. When effective oral progesterones were discovered, they changed society because their development paved the way for the development of the birth control pill. These orally administered, progesterone-like substances are called progestins (progestogens).

If you want to check out which type of hormone you are taking, read the label on the bottle or the descriptive leaflet inside the package. The manufacturer usually prints the trade name in large letters with the generic, or chemical, name in smaller letters below it. Sometimes you can save money by buying equivalent, but lower-priced, generic substitutes. Before you do, however, be aware that not all manufacturing processes are the same, and before you substitute one product for another, consult your physician. In describing these hormones in this chapter, we have used their generic chemical names, not their trade names. (For a complete listing of brands, refer to the tables in appendix A, which list the various estrogens and progestins both by their generic and trade names as well as the dosages that are available and the way they can be administered.)

Differences between Progesterone and Progestin

They sound alike, but they are quite different. Progesterone is the natural hormone that your ovary produces. The synthetic hormones, usually derived from male hormones that function like progesterone, we call either progestins or progestogens.

Using progestin as part of postmenopausal hormone treatment came into vogue following the estrogen/cancer controversy in the 1970s. Until a few years ago, we thought that there were few harmful effects caused by progestin use after menopause. Progestin also was thought to work only when taken along with estrogen. This belief changed when medical science realized that the progestins were quite potent hormones that also acted alone. Moreover, evidence began to indicate that progestins might increase a woman's risk of heart disease and breast disease. Nothing is yet conclusive, but this new knowledge has caused doctors to give much greater attention to which brand of progestin they use and what dose they prescribe.

Different Ways to Take HRT

HRT can be taken in a variety of ways. There are advantages and disadvantages to each of the different methods.

Pills

The most often prescribed and easiest method of taking HRT is via a tablet or capsule. This traditional method of taking the drug can create a problem. After you swallow the pill, the hormone enters the stomach and intestine, where it is absorbed into the circulatory system that leads to the liver. A problem can occur because the hormone undergoes change within the bowel before absorption and is absorbed as an altered substance with either reduced potency or different effects. Once transported directly to the liver in large amounts, the hormone can again be changed by the liver. It can also stimulate various actions in the liver itself, some potentially good and some possibly harmful. Either way, the hormone, metabolized in the liver, enters the general circulation of the body and begins to work. Its benefits and risks depend on whether its composition was changed in the liver and to what degree.

Shots (Intramuscular Injections)

One method of bypassing the liver is to inject the hormone directly into the muscle. The hormone can be mixed into other substances that will cause it to absorb into the system slowly, which helps to lengthen the intervals between shots from daily to once a month. There are some disadvantages to this method. The main one is that there is a high level of hormones in the blood shortly after the injection, which diminishes over time. Thus, there is an imbalance in the treatment's overall benefit, because there may be too much hormone in the blood right after the shot is administered and too little later in the cycle. At present, shots cannot be spaced more than a month apart, and some women find that having to go to the doctor's office to get an injection that often is disadvantageous because of the extra expenditure of time and money.

Implants (Subcutaneous Pellets)

Implants were popular in the 1960s and 1970s. They are outdated today. Since they may return in a new form, you should know how they work. The hormone combines with a solid material and is shaped into a pellet. The physician inserts the pellet into the subcutaneous fat through a small incision in the woman's lower abdominal wall or the top of her buttock. The pellets dissolve slowly and the hormone is absorbed through the fatty tissue. Over the years, there were many different strengths and mixtures of hormones used as implants. There are potential disadvantages. First, they may be difficult to remove, if removal becomes necessary because of possible side effects such as infection at the site of insertion. Further, the lifespan of the implant is capricious, so it is very difficult to know how long they will work and when they should be replaced. Research is underway to create better release mechanisms for implants, and it is likely that implants will be one of the practicable methods of the future.

Vaginal Creams (Vaginal Application)

Hormones can be applied directly to the vaginal area. Virtually all the estrogens listed in appendix A are available as creams for this purpose. Women who experience localized vaginal discomforts, such as dryness or itching, can obtain relief with this method. When women take estrogen vaginally, the hormone is absorbed through the vaginal epithelium into the blood system, which can be an advantage if the estrogen is needed, or a disadvantage if they should not be taking estrogen anyway, as is the case with women who have breast cancer and who therefore are not candidates for HRT. Because of this absorption, vaginal creams are not prescribed for women who should not take estrogen, but they can even be a problem for women who can take estrogen. These creams are impractical, because the amount of estrogen absorbed is so variable and the body may absorb too much.

Patches and Creams (Transdermal Systems)

Research in France in the early 1970s led to a breakthrough in the understanding of the absorption of hormones. It proved that estrogen creams rubbed onto the skin would be absorbed easily, enter into the circulatory system, and work well. The result is the availability of two newer ways to replace estrogen: a cream and a transdermal, or through-the-skin, patch.

The percutaneous cream contains specific strengths of hormones to be applied over a specified area of the body. In this way, a specific dose of the hormone can be administered on a daily basis. The hormone gets into the circulatory system without going through the liver so that the side effects generated by liver metabolism can be avoided. One disadvantage is that it can be messy. Moreover, a woman may accidentally vary the amount of skin she covers when applying the cream, which would result in a dose that is different one day from the next. Or the cream could be rubbed off before it is fully absorbed, with the same poor result.

Interestingly, there were early complaints by male partners of women using these creams because the men began to notice breast growth in themselves! This growth was presumably from couples lying close together and the cream accidentally being rubbed onto the man's chest. The newer formulations of the cream have a rapid drying property that practically eliminates these rubbing-off and transfer problems.

Transdermal skin patches are the most recent breakthrough in estrogen therapy. These specially devised patches place estrogen directly on the surface of the skin without the messiness or uneven coverage/dosage of creams. The patches are similar in appearance to those that heart patients wear containing ever-ready nitroglycerin. The estrogen transdermal patch is a multilayered system. Beneath an outer impermeable layer of plastic lies a reservoir of estrogen dissolved in alcohol, covered by a layer of permeable plastic.

This design is ingenious: It prevents the estrogen from seeping through the outside of the patch, while permitting it to seep inside to the skin, which gradually absorbs it. A ring of adhesive holds the patch onto the skin. The amount of estrogen given to a woman can be controlled by the size of the patch and the amount of estrogen that is inside the reservoir. These quarter-sized patches must be changed twice each week, every three to four days, so that they deliver a constant amount of estrogen. Women change these quickly themselves. They are worn on the hip, upper thigh, or lower abdomen.

One disadvantage of the patch is that it may irritate the skin under it, which is a problem for about one in twenty women. This problem can often be alleviated by moving the patch to a new spot on the skin each time a new one is applied. The advantage of the patch and the skin cream is the ease with which the doctor can check the amount of estrogen in the blood at subsequent follow-up visits to fine-tune the dosage to meet the needs of each individual woman.

Finding the Right Treatment Regimen

There have been many changes in the way we prescribe estrogens and progestins. These methods are referred to by doctors as *treatment regimens* or *treatment protocols.* They range from taking the hormones alone to taking them in various combinations with another hormone; from taking them continuously to receiving treatment in cycles that involve time on and off the medication. Learning about the various regimens and why and how we select them can help you understand why you may be taking hormones every day, whereas your best friend takes them cyclically.

Cyclic Regimen

Estrogen used alone, either cyclically or continuously, has been associated with an increase in the risk of uterine cancer. For this reason, we add progesterone or progestin. (The progestin inhibits the growth stimulation of estrogen.) The combination of estrogen and progestin, taken cyclically, is the most popular method of HRT today.

The cyclic treatment most frequently prescribed works in accord with the calendar month. You take estrogen from the first through the twenty-fifth day of the cycle, adding progestin for the last twelve or thirteen days of the estrogen therapy, and then stop both medications for the final days of the month. Withdrawal bleeding may occur at the end of the month during the pill-free days.

There are three cyclic methods popularly in use in the United States today:

- You take estrogen tablets on days one to twenty-five of the month and add progestin for approximately twelve days (days fourteen to twenty-five).
- You use the estrogen patch, changing it twice weekly for twenty-five days and take oral progestin on days fourteen to twenty-five.
- You take one of the other estrogens and progestins in equivalent doses and cycle twenty-one days on and seven days off therapy. (These are listed in appendix A.)

These methods have one thing in common: About two-thirds of those women who have their uterus intact will experience a period during the treatment-free days. The amount of bleeding usually lessens over time and, after several years, may disappear altogether.

Continuous Therapy

Continuous therapy involves the uninterrupted use of estrogen. Recent prescribing trends have moved away from the interrupted, or cycled, use of estrogen, which actually rests on little scientific foundation.

Continuous estrogen with intermittent progestin has become the most popular U.S. method of continuous therapy. It works this way: You take estrogen continuously, either as a daily tablet or as a skin patch changed twice each week. You take progestin on the first twelve days of the calendar month.

More than two-thirds of women with an intact uterus will, on this regimen, experience bleeding. Bleeding, however, should occur only after the twelfth day when the progestin is stopped and last until around the sixteenth day. If bleeding occurs before the ninth of the month, it may suggest that the dose of the progestin is too low and should be adjusted. Bleeding starting after the sixteenth day should be considered irregular and reported to your physician.

Combined Continuous Therapy

Combined continuous therapy is a more innovative method of hormone replacement. This therapy involves daily doses of estrogen combined with low daily doses of progestin. The combined continuous method attempts to avoid that most unpopular side effect of HRT, *withdrawal bleeding,* that usually occurs with cyclic therapy. Variable results of this therapy have been reported in recent medical literature.

Dr. Utian's personal experience with women using this form of therapy is that they have irregular bleeding during the first six months of treatment. Endometrial sampling (biopsy) is often required, which generally shows a mixed pattern of estrogen and progestin in the uterine lining. Most women do not like the irregular bleeding and stop taking therapy. Those who continue usually find that they stop bleeding after approximately six months.

Is it worth it? Further research is necessary in order to answer this question. It seems likely that this form of combined continuous therapy may become very popular in the future. The main hesitation in prescribing it now is the risk of giving the body too much progestin, with a possible risk of heart disease or breast disease as a result.

Continuous Progestin Therapy

Progestin only, taken continuously, is a form of therapy for women who cannot take estrogen because they have had breast or uterine cancer, or because they have severe fibrocystic breast disease. Women take it either daily in pill form or in monthly intramuscular shots.

Progestins help to prevent osteoporosis. Their protection of bone, however, is not as good as that of estrogen. The major disadvantage of progestin-only therapy is that it may increase the risk of heart disease.

Finding the Right Dosages of HRT

The amount of medication you take is determined by your specific need for and response to treatment. For example, if you require short-term relief of minor symptoms, you take as low a dose as possible, which may be increased if necessary.

A good rule of thumb is that you should take the lowest possible dose that can bring you the relief you desire. According to FDA recommendation, you should take it for the shortest possible time. But how is the lowest effective dose estimated? Medical scientists have studied this question for years and discovered many ways to assess a woman's response to treatment. These include relief of symptoms, changes in the appearance of vaginal cells (seen in a test called hormonal cytology), and increases of blood hormone levels, specifically the estrogen level. Repeated bone density tests, too, will show whether the therapy is protecting your bone.

There is a standardized dose that works for most women. Your individual dose should be determined over a period of time between you and your physician.

Hormones are potent medications, so do not change the dose of your hormone yourself. Always consult your physician about making any change in the course of your treatment. You can cause yourself such severe side effects as heavy bleeding, high blood pressure, and many other problems by altering your dosage. These will be discussed in more detail in chapter 6, when we weigh risk-to-benefit ratios of the various treatments.

HRT Treatment for Women Without a Uterus

The woman who has undergone a hysterectomy is decidedly at an advantage with HRT. She does not need to take progestin, which usually is prescribed because it reduces the risk of uterine cancer. However, there is no evidence that the progestins provide similar protection for the breast, and they may actually increase the risk of heart attack and breast cancer. So if you have had a hysterectomy, you can avoid the potential risks and side effects of progestin while you appreciate the benefits of estrogen therapy.

What to Expect During HRT

We have provided a full description of what to expect when you visit your physician in chapter 6. Still, it bears mentioning here that once you are undergoing treatment, you should anticipate regular visits to your physician.

At your follow-up visit, expect to give another detailed medical history relating to any changes in your symptoms, side effects, or any other problems that have developed in relation to your therapy. Your blood pressure should be measured and a general examination including your breasts and abdomen should be done at each visit. Pelvic examinations should be performed annually and a Pap smear should be done every one to two years.

Often, the question arises of whether or not to take an endometrial sampling (endometrial biopsy) as a means of screening for uterine cancer or correcting hormone dose. I feel that if you are taking your progestin in an adequate dose, and your bleeding pattern is normal, there is no reason for doing an annual sampling. However, if you are one of those women who take estrogen only, who have their uterus intact, and who do not take progestin for some specific reason (some women with their uterus intact refuse progestin because of its side effects), I would recommend having an endometrial sample every year. You should also anticipate having a baseline mammogram taken when you first begin therapy and an annual mammogram thereafter.

It is my recommendation that once you start HRT, you visit your physician at least every six months. If the examinations listed above are done, and no problems occur in the interim, you need only those biannual visits. However, if you experience any side effects such as breakthrough bleeding, you should report them to your physician and anticipate that an endometrial sample may be taken.

It is also important that your doctor closely monitor the amount of estrogen you are taking and its effects on you. This monitoring may require testing your blood estrogen levels and measuring your calcium levels to assure that you are not losing calcium, which can lead to losing bone. One way of determining calcium levels is with the *urine calcium creatinine test*. Bone density testing, explained in chapter 3, is a method of determining bone loss that is very important for women at risk for osteoporosis. It shows whether bone mass has been maintained or improved with therapy. If bone density test results show that bone loss is continuing, then the method and/or type of HRT should be changed.

Current Trends and Future Directions for HRT

All the latest research on HRT still has not told us everything that we need to know medically. Large national studies in the United States and elsewhere are racing to fill in the gaps. Researchers are studying the effects of the specific types of estrogen, their dosages, the treatment regimens, and the proper mixture of estrogen with other hormones. More scientific information will be forthcoming, although current thought continues to favor HRT.

You can expect future methods of taking hormones to include new implant systems and new creams, and also that new types of hormones will be discovered.

Nonhormonal Medications

Although your body responds best to hormones and should be treated with them, if possible, nonhormonal drugs can play a role in offering relief from midlife discomforts. If you cannot take hormones for the reasons outlined below, however, there are other means of treatment that can be considered. We want to offer a word of caution here. It is important that you and your doctor investigate any symptoms that you have to try to learn their specific causes. If you have symptoms that may be caused by psychological or sociocultural factors, perhaps they ought to be treated with an educational or a psychosocial therapeutic approach. In such a case, drugs would be an adjunct to other forms of therapy.

It is important as well that you receive treatment that is symptom-specific. Be careful with yourself. Don't assume that all the symptoms that you have are related to menopause just because you are experiencing menopause. Guided by your own introspection, and by the results of clinical tests, work with your physician to decide what's what!

Even though nonhormonal drugs are not primary sources of relief for menopausal discomforts, your doctor might advise you to take them in the following situations:

- If you cannot use HRT for medical reasons
- If you do not get relief from HRT
- If you do not want HRT, but do want symptom relief
- If you cannot tolerate HRT because of side effects, such as nausea or fluid retention

It can be difficult to select the right nonhormonal drug for the treatment of climacteric problems. Often the physician's choice rests more on guesswork than on the proven effects of treatment, as there are not enough studies that document conclusively the therapeutic efficacy of nonhormonal drugs.

As editor of the medical publication *Maturitas,* Dr. Utian analyzed the articles published over an eight-year span and discovered that more than 90 percent were about the use of hormones compared to fewer than 10 percent about the efficacy of nonhormonal medications. Further, in nine out of ten of the articles on nonhormonal medications, physicians reported more side effects than benefits with these medications. Although very few nonhormonal medications currently available effectively combat climacteric syndrome problems such as hot flashes, some may work, and you should be aware of them.

There are seven kinds of nonhormonal medications. They include the following:

- Sedatives (for sleep)
- Tranquilizers (to induce calmness)
- Antidepressants
- Clonidine
- Propranolol
- Vitamin B$_6$ (pyridoxine)
- Vitamin E

Sedatives may reduce the number of hot flashes you endure, but are less helpful in relieving irritability and emotional upset. Phenobarbital USP, alone or in combination with other drugs, seems to be effective and is available commercially as Bellergal tablets. However, sedatives are less effective than HRT in reducing menopause problems.

Tranquilizers comprise a large group of drugs that are often abused in the care of postmenopausal women when they are prescribed before HRT. When chosen as an appropriate treatment method, monitored, and used with educational and psychotherapeutic programs—only if the "agitated states" are not biologically caused—they are helpful for women with excessive anxiety, irritability, insomnia, and related agitated states. The most often prescribed tranquilizers are Valium, Librium, Ativan, Xanax, Buspar, and some of the phenothiazines.

Antidepressants are prescribed for the same reasons as tranquilizers; however, they are used in cases of severe depression. Among the most commonly used are Elavil, Nardil, Parnate, Sinequan, and Tofranil.

Clonidine has received attention because of its helpfulness in combating hot flashes. At first, it was manufactured in low dose as an antimigraine drug; and later it was made in high dose as an antihypertensive drug. Then, doctors reported that it appeared to reduce perimenopausal flushing. Some studies support this observation; others do not, but there is reason to hope that further research will find a nonhormonal treatment for hot flashes.

Propranolol (Inderal) is another drug that was studied for its effect on hot flashes, but it has not been found effective.

Vitamin B_6 is sometimes suggested, because there is some evidence that the loss of sex hormones may cause a deficiency in this vitamin. Symptoms of such deficiency may include depression, emotional instability, fatigue, disturbances in concentration, and loss of libido. These symptoms may respond to 50–200 milligrams of vitamin B_6 taken daily. Do not take megadoses: The side effects may include altered tryptophan metabolism (tryptophan is the amino acid that maintains normal nitrogen equilibrium in the body), which can be worse than the original problem.

Vitamin E, taken in megadoses, has gathered more than its share of claims for the relief of hot flashes. Many women claim relief, yet with careful comparative testing the vitamin did not pass the effectiveness test. As with other substances, anything taken in excess is risky business. I do not recommend megadoses of vitamin E, because liver problems may result.

Making the Most of HRT and Nonhormonal Therapy

As you continue reading this book, it will become apparent that you should not rely entirely on hormones or other medications to enhance the quality of life after menopause. It is within your power to take very practical measures that can prevent or alleviate many of the symptoms that occur.

For example, there is a natural approach to take against osteoporosis. Remember that osteoporosis is preventable if you can control two main processes. First, you can develop as much bone as possible during your first forty years, before menopause. Second, you can reduce the rate of bone loss that may occur after menopause.

Success in doing these things often requires some changes in lifestyle that call for dedication and persistence. But, studies have shown conclusively that an inappropriate diet, lack of weight-bearing exercise, and heavy cigarette smoking contribute to loss of bone. If you are willing to make a few changes in your lifestyle, you could protect your skeleton. To help you, we offer the Menopause Dietstyle in chapter 7 and explore specific exercise options in chapter 8.

There is still the problem of hot flashes and the question of whether they can be alleviated without drugs. Hot flashes are one of the most disabling symptoms of menopause. They can interfere with the quality of a woman's life and even with her ability to function. There is no doubt that HRT remains the most effective method known for dealing with this symptom.

For women who cannot tolerate taking estrogens, or who are not medically permitted to take HRT, the fact that nonhormonal medications are not generally effective can be a desperate medical dilemma. Biofeedback training may provide some relief in such cases. With this process women learn to control and manipulate various body mechanisms, such as heart rate, blood vessel diameter, and muscle tension, which are usually controlled without your awareness by your autonomous nervous system. Research in biofeedback training is still in its early stages, but we hope that in the future it may offer a nonpharmacologic means of reducing the discomfort of hot flashes.

Work continues as well with progressive relaxation training, a fairly recent method for learning how to relieve stress and tension through practiced relaxation, which may bring some relief. While new techniques are under study, you can try other minor changes in your lifestyle to reduce the severity or the number of your hot flashes. Changing the kind of clothes you wear may help. Give up heavy sweaters and try layering clothing instead. Alter your activities whenever possible to reduce stress. Attempting to gain some conscious control of your hot flashes through relaxation therapy may be productive. A good relaxation therapist can teach you how.

Avoiding Cardiovascular Disease

As we will discuss later, the use of estrogen in HRT does appear to be associated with a distinct reduction in the risk of cardiovascular disease. Other factors can also be employed to reduce the incidence of this disease. We write about them in detail in chapters 7 and 8.

Other ways of combating heart disease without estrogen include stopping smoking. Smoking is the most harmful of all habits and probably the most significant cause of coronary heart disease. Another method is gaining control of the stresses in your life and working toward reducing your negative responses to them if you cannot eliminate the stresses themselves.

Enhanced Well-Being

An early finding of Dr. Utian's work—and the first medical report of such finding—was that estrogen therapy offered an enhanced feeling of general well-being. Although estrogen does not act chemically as an antidepressant, it certainly enhances mood. It has a "mental tonic effect."

Exercise also produces this special feeling of well-being. Often termed "runner's euphoria" or "swimmer's high," athletes sometimes cite this sense of well-being as one of the benefits of pursuing their sport. Many people start an exercise program, lose interest, and drop out. Quitting is most likely to occur during the first three months of an exercise program, which is a shame, because most studies show that the mood-enhancing effects of exercise develop strongly after three months of regular exercise. After several months, you usually achieve physical fitness as well. If you hang in there, you can expect to feel better, enjoy all of your activities more, combat exhaustion from work, and perhaps relieve menopausal discomforts. The benefits of and suggestions for exercise programs that work are outlined in chapter 8.

Diagnosing the Climacteric

You may want to know how your doctor diagnoses your entry into the climacteric. It is difficult to confirm, if you have not yet become menopausal. There are some telltale symptoms, however, such as changes in your menstrual pattern and the onset of hot flashes, which offer diagnostic clues.

We suspect menopause when there is a long interval without periods in a woman over the age of fifty, particularly if she has hot flashes or a low estrogen profile. The low estrogen profile can be discovered during a physical examination by means of an atrophic vaginal smear, the absence of vaginal mucus, or an atrophic endometrium, diagnosed by a biopsy.

In younger women, if the menses have been absent for one year, there may be a strong reason to diagnose menopause. FSH levels in the blood can be measured, and if they are elevated, then you are beyond menopause. Ideally, you should not wait this long without a period before seeking medical advice.

Diagnostic difficulties can come from several sources. When a woman in her thirties or forties loses her period, she is often referred to a gynecologic endocrine unit to search for reasons other than premature menopause. Another diagnostic challenge arises when an older woman on oral contraceptives asks if she can stop taking the pill without fear of pregnancy. Answering this question requires that she stop the pill and then have her FSH levels monitored before she can be assured that ovulation has, indeed, stopped. After hysterectomy, hot flashes are the most frequent signal of menopause, but the diagnosis of menopause is conclusively determined by measurement of the FSH levels in the blood.

Once menopause is confirmed, and if hormones are prescribed, you must see your gynecologist at least once every six months. This schedule is important to assess your general health and to determine your response to HRT, if you are taking it. It is up to you to assure your continued good health and fitness by following the treatment program that you and your gynecologist devise. If you are under any other physician's treatment, you should visit that physician twice a year, in addition to your gynecologist. Be sure that each doctor knows what the other is prescribing or recommending for you, so that they both can work together to bring you maximum benefits.

·6·

Choices and Chances:
Are Hormone Treatments
Right for You?

"Should I take hormones?"
  "Are hormones dangerous?"
  "Does estrogen cause uterine cancer?"
  "Does progestin increase my risk of breast cancer?"
  "How do I gain a perspective about the risks and the benefits?"
  These questions are serious and cannot be answered with a simple "yes" or "no." They call into question how you live your life. Life is an interesting business. It is filled with good things and it is filled with risks. We enjoy life and balance it by practicing the *minimax concept.*

Every day you engage in activities that entail risk, yet you undertake these activities because of some advantage that they offer you. Some things are ordinary; others bring excitement or challenge into your life. For example, you may be fearful of terrorists or of the safety of aging airplanes, but you choose to board a flight from New York to Athens. You repeatedly hear that aspirin can cause stomach ulcers, but you take it anyway to relieve a painful injury. Every day you make many decisions, and with each you weigh, consciously or unconsciously, the risk and the benefit of your action. If your calculations demonstrate that a given course of action entails too much risk for your peace of mind, you don't move ahead with it. If the risks seem minimal, or worth the projected gains, you proceed. Thus, you attempt to maximize your benefits and minimize your risks.

The Minimax Concept and HRT

Balance is an important ingredient in the good life. Balancing the risks against the benefits is how you decide whether to start long-term hormonal therapy.

You must understand the full range of risks and benefits of post-menopausal hormone therapy. In this chapter, we will present the facts so that you can weigh HRT on your own risk/benefit scales to arrive at your decision. HRT is, ultimately, your choice.

How do you feel about reading articles headlined "Estrogens Double Breast Cancer Risks" and "Estrogens Prevent Heart Attacks" in the same week? Confused? Then use the minimax concept to weigh risks against benefits.

We cannot deny that major issues need to be considered when you assess the value of HRT. There are so many factors that influence the therapy: nutrition, exercise, smoking, the use and abuse of drugs and alcohol, and even other prescribed medications. It's complicated. Take the following as an example. A sedentary fifty-eight-year-old woman begins an exercise program that improves her cardiovascular system, improves her muscular strength and her endurance, makes her more flexible and perhaps even decreases her risk of fractures because of her added bone mass and increased coordination, and enhances the quality of her life. But what if she started the exercise program at approximately the same time that she began HRT? How does she weigh the contribution of exercise and hormone therapy in assessing the improvement to the quality of her life? The question is only important if she is trying to decide to give up one of these activities.

What about smoking? There is a dramatic relationship between smoking and heart disease. If a woman stops smoking, and takes hormones and feels better, what worked? Both actions? How does she weigh each in terms of its value to her life? Again, she might only question her choices if she is considering giving up HRT, for whatever reason, or wants to resume smoking.

Benefits of HRT

What can you gain from HRT? Below is a list of the benefits that HRT may bring you:

Enhance quality of life
  Mental tonic effect
  Improved sleep
  Improved short-term memory
Prevent osteoporosis and fractures
Prevent heart attack
Eliminate hot flashes
Enhance sexuality
  Enhanced sensation
  Increased buildup of vaginal epithelium
  Improved pelvic floor muscles
Slower overall body deterioration
  Smoother skin
  Tauter bladder/pelvic floor muscle tone
  Firmer breasts
  Improved muscle tone
Increase longevity

Sounds good, doesn't it? So if you're an appropriate candidate for HRT, which you and your gynecologist ultimately will decide together, put these factors on the plus side of the scale.

Downside of HRT

Below is a list of risk factors associated with HRT. Study it carefully:

Potential minor problems
  Uterovaginal bleeding
  Breast tenderness
  PMS-like symptoms
  Some inconvenience and cost
Potential major problems
  Uterine cancer
  Breast cancer
Blood clots
Gallstones
Hypertension
Surgery

Balancing the Risks and the Benefits

Now you've got a group of features on each side of your scale. Before you balance it, remember that you are seeking the right balance for *you*. If you already have major risk factors, as described in chapter 5, it is likely that the risks will outweigh the benefits. If you are the average woman, with relatively few risk factors, the advantages will far outweigh the risks.

Minor Side Effects of HRT
Although most women respond well to HRT taken as described in chapter 5, there can be side effects. They range from minor nuisances to major problems. Most of the nuisances disappear within a few months after you start therapy, enabling most women to gain the full benefits of HRT.

Vaginal bleeding after menopause is a real disadvantage of post-menopausal estrogen therapy. Whether or not you bleed may be determined by the hormone selected for you, the dose you take, the dosing regimen, and your unique response to therapy (see appendix A). There are many women who fear a connection between post-menopausal bleeding and cancer. If you feel this way, perhaps you should eliminate this cause for anxiety and either discuss and allay your fears or elect not to take HRT.

After menopause, the normal decrease in estrogen results in the thinning of your uterine lining. As a result, your periods stop. When estrogen is brought back into your system through HRT, the lining thickens again. If you are on a cyclic regimen, when you stop taking the hormone, during the last days of the cycle, the tissue of the lining loses its nourishment, thins, and is shed as menstrual flow. If you are not on hormones, any bleeding from the vagina that occurs six months or longer after menopause is called postmenopausal bleeding. Consider it a signal that something may be wrong. Never ignore post-menopausal bleeding. Consult with your doctor. The bleeding may be the early warning of uterine cancer, or it may represent nothing of significance. Let your physician decide.

On hormone therapy, the bleeding you may experience is called withdrawal bleeding, which occurs when the hormones, particularly progestin, are withdrawn from your treatment. This bleeding is normal. However, breakthrough bleeding, which may occur while you are still on estrogen and progestin, should be reported to your physician.

Research is underway to find new ways for taking the hormone cyclically that will either reduce or eliminate the bleeding. Meanwhile, withdrawal bleeding, although it is a nuisance, is not in itself a sound reason for not taking estrogen.

Breast pain may result from HRT, especially if you add progestin to your estrogen treatment. You may experience swollen or tender breasts. Rarely is the pain so severe that your medication needs to be changed or stopped. This condition is called *mastalgia* and is similar to the breast tenderness that some women of reproductive age feel before the onset of their menstrual periods. It is caused by the domino-like effect of the added progestin on the estrogen on the tissue cells in the breast, which may cause a slight amount of vascular congestion or fluid retention within the breast itself. It is not a pleasant symptom and it can be difficult to prevent.

To alleviate other contributors to breast swelling, most physicians will recommend simple dietary changes such as reducing your intake of salt as well as coffee, chocolate, and other substances containing caffeine and xanthine (tissue- and heart-stimulating substances). Small doses of vitamin B_6 may also be of value in reducing mastalgia. Once in a while, if the problem is severe, a mild diuretic may be prescribed. If none of these methods work, the hormone therapy may have to be discontinued and then started again at a lower dose, especially the progestin.

Other PMS-like symptoms that may appear during the first few months of HRT include slight swelling of the legs, an increase in body weight, nausea, and even minor depression. (Depression is more the result of the progestin than estrogen.) Although some of these symptoms may be related to mild water retention (edema), it is generally best to persist with the treatment until your body creates its own balance. Diuretics, in my opinion, are not recommended medically because they can introduce their own set of problems for you.

Weight gain with HRT often is the result of fluid retention. If you gain weight, but are not retaining fluid, you are probably eating too much. Hormones can make you hungrier. Use the Dietstyle in chapter 7 to exert greater dietary control while getting the nutrients you need.

The solutions for reducing these PMS-like symptoms are similar to those described for breast tenderness. They include reducing salt intake, avoiding caffeine- and xanthine-containing products, trying vitamin B_6, plus increasing physical activities and exercise. If your symptoms are particularly severe, your physician may reduce your dose of the progestin or try a different progestin. In most instances, the manipulation of the medications is successful and reduces the nuisance symptoms without affecting the advantages of HRT.

Medication inconvenience may be a new thought for you, even though you know that you sometimes forget to take your medicine on time, or at all. Some women prefer taking medicine by mouth and have an easy time remembering to take their tablets daily. Others find the skin patches more convenient and appreciate the presence of the patch on their bodies because it acts as a medication reminder to change the patch twice a week.

Treatment cost is another inconvenience. It involves three components: the physician visits, the repeated laboratory and special-test charges, and the cost of the drugs themselves. There are clearcut advantages to taking the therapy, such as spending money now to ensure wellness later, since illness later could be more expensive. Regrettably, most health insurers and reimbursers are not yet convinced of the value of preventive healthcare and continue to prefer to pay only for crisis medicine. Perhaps you should help lobby for preventive healthcare coverage!

Inasmuch as you are responsible for the costs, once you are on a satisfactory program of HRT, you can usually save money by purchasing your hormones in three- to six-month batches. You may want to check into the value of generic drugs. Check with your physician before substituting!

Potential Major Problems
You must be fully alert to the potential risks that could be serious, so you can detect their early warning signs. Your awareness may significantly reduce the likelihood of any of them becoming real risks to you.

Uterine cancer was not considered a viable risk until late 1975, although warnings linking it with estrogen replacement therapy appeared in early medical publications, including one of my own. In 1968, I wrote, "These potent hormones should ideally not be administered by medical practitioners in the absence of definite climacteric symptoms until there is clearer evidence of the relationship between the development of carcinoma and the administration of estrogens."

In December 1975, two articles appeared in the *New England Journal of Medicine* stating that estrogen treatment seemed to be associated with an increased risk of uterine cancer. This research triggered the bitter estrogen debate, which is reflected in a prodigious amount of medical literature. Many details of this medical debate appeared in print. Only recently have sufficient research findings enabled doctors to apply some perspective to the situation.

Following the flurry of debate about estrogen's harmful effects, which continues today, the FDA decided that the evidence was strong enough to hold several inquiries. It ordered a warning to be printed on every estrogen-containing product on the market. Meanwhile, the question still requires an answer: Just how great is the risk?

The chance of developing uterine cancer after menopause is about one in every thousand women per year. The risk of uterine cancer to women on estrogen therapy depends on how high the dose is and for how long it is taken. The worst scenario is that the cancer risk increases to between four and eight women in every thousand per year. Thus, estrogen may increase risk of uterine cancer from four to eight times. The majority of these estrogen-induced cases of uterine cancer are of low virulence, however, and can be successfully cured if caught at an early stage. The death rates from uterine cancer have declined every year since 1930. There was no increase in death rates during the 1960s and 1970s when estrogens were prescribed in high doses. To gain additional perspective, consider that smoking just twenty cigarettes a day increases the risk of death from lung cancer by seventeen times.

Taking all this information into consideration, what follows is the best advice that we can give in answer to the question, Should I take HRT? Estrogen therapy, without progestin, does carry a risk for a woman who has her uterus intact. When progestin is added, this increased risk is negated. The modern way of prescribing estrogen, in low doses and with cycled progestin, makes the risk of uterine cancer small. Yet you must be aware that if you have other risk factors, such as obesity, abnormal uterine bleeding, a family history of cancer, and, possibly, cigarette smoking, the individual risk to you is increased.

If you are on HRT, you must commit yourself to consulting your physician for problems as they occur and to follow-up office visits every six months. At these visits, breast and pelvic examinations and cancer screening tests, if required, should be done.

It is up to you to report any unusual bleeding. Your doctor is as aware as you are of the potential dangers and the respect that HRT demands. Finally, the answer to your question is that the scientific evidence to date does not indicate that HRT should be stopped.

Breast cancer and its relationship to hormone therapy is a more cloudy issue. There have been at least twenty important studies in the last decade that explored the use of postmenopausal hormones and the development of breast cancer. Most of them show no increased risk or reduced risk of breast cancer with therapy. One study did show a slight increase in risk in patients who take estrogen by injection, but otherwise it demonstrates no risk related to the dose or the duration of other methods of estrogen therapy. Three studies show a slight increase in risk. The nature of the risk was an increase from one case per thousand per year to 1.2 cases per thousand per year following twelve years of continuous estrogen use, and two cases per thousand after twenty years of continuous use.

The most recent study on breast cancer risk appeared in the *New England Journal of Medicine* on August 3, 1989. In it, the risk appeared to be increased to 1.7 times that for the general population—still not a dramatic increase. Yet, it does suggest an increase in risk rather than confirming our thinking that the combination of estrogen and progestin would decrease the risk of breast cancer. To quote from the editorial that accompanied that article, "The data are not conclusive enough to warrant any immediate change in the way we [doctors] approach hormone replacement, but they do show the need for additional research."

It is reassuring that there has been no increase in the number of deaths from breast cancer over the last fifty years. It follows that estrogen and progestin therapy does not seem to increase the death rate. Unfortunately, there is almost no decrease in the rate of breast cancer deaths, either.

The general medical consensus today is that women with an intact uterus should take progestin with their estrogen. Estrogen can be taken alone if the uterus is absent, since the addition of progestin does not seem to protect the breasts, and is obviously not needed to protect the uterus in this case. In all instances, the strong recommendation is for an annual mammogram while on HRT and a semiannual breast examination by a physician, in addition to breast self-examination. As an added plus, the development of any breast problems that are unrelated to HRT will be diagnosed earlier as well.

Early evidence suggested that the risk of blood clots was increased in postmenopausal women under two circumstances. One was in the group of women using synthetic estrogens (ethinyl estradiol and mestranol) and the other was in the group of women who smoke. The number of deaths from blood clots for women taking the birth control pill are normally quoted at about 4 to 6 deaths per 100,000 women per year. In applying the minimax principle, place this statistic against the 35 in 100,000 people likely to die each year on our highways.

Let's consider the risk factors associated with an increased chance of developing blood clots. These include obesity, high blood pressure, cigarette smoking, severe varicose veins, and a previous history of thrombosis. Have you noticed how often smoking and obesity appear as risk factors? Is it time for you to quit smoking? Is it also time for you to begin the Menopause Dietstyle described in chapter 7?

Studies have been done to determine whether taking estrogens will affect the clotting substances in the blood. These showed that the types of estrogens used in treating the postmenopause do not seem to alter blood coagulation factors significantly. Recent studies of hormones not taken by mouth have been even more reassuring. For example, in patients using estrogen skin patches, studies of blood-clotting factors show that these factors are unchanged.

At present, medical practice suggests that women with preexisting risk factors for blood clots should not take HRT. If there was only a single incidence several years in the past, it still is considered safe to prescribe HRT, although it may be preferable to use the skin patch rather than an oral medication.

Liver problems and gallstones must also be considered. Some pregnant women complain of itchy skin. It occurs because of the effect of high estrogen levels on the liver. This problem is most unusual with estrogen treatment, but it does prove that estrogen has an effect on the liver. For this reason, estrogen should not be taken by anyone with liver disorders.

A related report shows that women taking estrogens have a 2.5-time greater chance of developing gallstones requiring surgical treatment. Obesity is also associated with an increased incidence of gallstones. (Medical textbooks describe the classical presentation of a patient with an inflamed gallbladder as being a "female, fair, fat, and forty.")

In order to prevent gallbladder problems, it is important to reduce cholesterol in your diet, which also helps to prevent heart disease. Another safe way would be to use a form of estrogen replacement that does not involve the liver. The skin patch appears to have less influence on liver enzymes than oral estrogen and may reduce the incidence of gallstones, although there have been no confirmatory clinical studies to prove this theory.

Increased blood pressure, or hypertension, is often considered to be a reason for not taking HRT. Hypertension is known to increase the risk of heart attacks. Fortunately, there is general medical agreement that estrogenic hormones will not normally alter your blood pressure. So you can take HRT even if you are hypertensive. There are a very few patients who show an idiosyncratic response, which means they have an unusual response to medication. For women with an idiosyncratic response, their blood pressure increases shortly after starting on the oral estrogens.

Your follow-up examinations with your doctor will include having your blood pressure checked. If your blood pressure is elevated, the best advice is to switch from the pill to the patch. The patch will not affect the liver enzymes that elevate blood pressure.

Surgery can be one complication of taking hormones. It is a fact that HRT results in vaginal bleeding and, occasionally, in irregular bleeding, which may make you subject to more endometrial samplings (biopsy), diagnostic curettage, and perhaps even hysterectomy. The rate of hysterectomy in the United States is reported to have increased from 602 procedures per 100,000 women in 1970 to 727 procedures per 100,000 in 1975. Since then, the numbers have stayed about the same. What is not known is the influence, if any, of HRT on this statistical increase.

The newer, simpler techniques for endometrial sampling, as well as our improved understanding of the use of the progestins, should enable the medical profession to reduce a woman's risk for surgery. Nonetheless, you should be aware that the possibility for surgery does exist.

Improved Quality of Life

Should you consider taking HRT? Is there any advantage inherent in this form of therapy? The answer is an unequivocal "yes." When you weigh the results of the untreated climacteric against the minor and major problems that can evolve from HRT, the answer is "yes" for women who are appropriate candidates for therapy. The list of advantages of HRT is long and proven.

Improved quality of life and relief of symptoms is welcomed by most women. Quality of life cannot be quantified. Your mood, your feeling of well-being, and your satisfaction with yourself and your surroundings is perceived differently by you than it will be by other women. It is a very individual matter. Your societal and domestic status can also play a role in how you feel and react to menopause. Are you aware that some societies reward women for having reached menopause or the end of their fertile period, whereas other societies punish them? For example, women of the Rajput classes in India look forward to menopause because they emerge from *purdah* (veiled faces) at the end of their childbearing years. They can assume their positions as wise elders. On the other hand, a woman with hot flashes in a youth-oriented society may find little support or understanding of her transition through the climacteric.

The main trend revealed by studies of popular attitudes is that although some women in western societies have an overall negative image of menopause, this negative response is not as widespread as was previously thought. Today, the vast majority of women at midlife do not express regret at reaching menopause, do not report more symptoms or poorer health status, and do not increase their use of medical services. The negative attitudes that do exist appear to be the province of younger women and seem to be based on an outdated stereotype of the menopausal woman. (Men, however, are quite a different story and will be discussed in chapter 11.)

The typical menopausal woman today holds optimistic beliefs about maintaining her femininity and sexuality. Unfortunately, she may be confused about how to do that and what to expect. There is still little doubt that taking hormones after menopause does have direct beneficial effects on mood and behavior, and therefore on the quality of life.

Relief of Hot Flashes

The relief of hot flashes is the most significant benefit you will perceive soon after starting HRT. Estrogens are remarkably effective in eliminating this annoying symptom. Hot flashes can occur during the day or at night, as "night sweats," and can cause sleeping disturbance up to and including the need to shower, change night clothing, and change bedding. HRT brings relief from hot flashes and an improvement in sleep.

Improved Mental Outlook

The mental tonic effects of HRT were presumed for several years. In 1972, I reported the first definitive study that showed conclusively the mood-enhancing effects of estrogens on women who had lost ovarian function. Initially severely criticized by contemporary researchers, the findings in my study were confirmed within a few years by studies in Europe, the United Kingdom, and the United States.

The actual reasons for the mood-elevating effects are not fully understood, but it is known that estrogens have many effects within the brain and the nervous system. This mental tonic effect of estrogens, which is perceived as a feeling of overall well-being, goes beyond the fact that the hot flashes have been relieved. Women in my practice often describe a feeling of revitalization and of being reborn, which translates into better performance of daily duties and greater enjoyment of daily pleasures. These women feel more alert and better able to function.

Estrogens are not considered antidepressive drugs, but they may reduce minor depressions in some women. Major, continuing depression, however, is a different problem that requires different therapy.

In the late 1970s, studies at Harvard confirmed that estrogens enhanced the quality of sleep. We already knew that stopping the night sweats for women suffering hot flashes was likely to improve their sleep. This study showed that women without night sweats experienced an improvement in REM sleep (rapid eye movement—the good sleep). This improvement occurred for all the women on HRT. There was a deterioration of REM sleep in women deprived of HRT. Naturally, anyone who has a better night's sleep will feel better in the morning.

Improved Short-Term Memory
Improved short-term memory is a distinct advantage of HRT. We have often heard women around the age of menopause express concern because they "seem to be forgetting things." They can't remember the location of car keys, glasses, and so on, or they lose the tail-end of a thought when speaking or writing. We can usually blame some of these annoying situations on being busy and sometimes stressed at home or at work. So, a study from King's College Hospital, London, England, in the 1970s was surprising. It found a distinct difference in short-term memory between women who had active ovaries or were on postmenopausal HRT as compared to menopausal women without ovaries or HRT. These studies have been repeated, and continue to provide evidence that when women take estrogen their short-term memory improves.

Disease Prevention

Preventing osteoporosis is important. Ten years ago, osteoporosis was an unpronounceable and unintelligible word. Today it is in common use. Estrogen has been fully recognized as the single most important substance in the prevention of this crippling problem.

Preventing heart attacks has become the goal of both women and men now that we are all living longer. In chapter 3, we cited evidence that premature menopause is associated with an increased risk of *ischemic heart disease* (heart disease and heart attacks). Consequently, a woman who loses her ovaries early in life, either spontaneously or as a result of surgery (like Nancy in our first case study), is more likely to have a heart attack.

Even more important are new data showing that HRT protects women from heart attack, reducing their chances by 50 percent. There is one problem with this rosy scenario. The role of the added progestin is not clear. It is possible that if too much or the wrong kind of progestin is taken, the beneficial effect of the estrogen will be negated. There are many major studies underway worldwide that should clarify this situation, including a large study under the auspices of the U.S. National Institutes of Health in Washington, D.C. This area of inquiry urgently requires an answer. Meanwhile, remember that there are many other things you can do to prevent heart attack, including appropriate exercise, careful nutrition, and no smoking.

Enhanced Sexuality

Estrogen is called the female hormone for good reason. The absence of it reduces sexuality whereas its presence enhances it. There are many ways in which estrogen can produce increased awareness, sensuality, desire, and enjoyment of sexual activity. We discuss these benefits in chapter 9.

Slowing Down the Aging Process

Slower overall body deterioration is every woman's objective. Estrogens cannot prevent aging. Time passes and we age. However, estrogen unquestionably slows the aging processes of your body. Let's look at how it works on the skin.

The skin is the largest organ of the body. It undergoes many changes related to menopause and has many responses to HRT. After menopause, it is not unusual for women to notice that their skin is thinner, dryer, and that their body hair begins to fall out. These changes are often reversible once you begin HRT. Within six months, your skin can appear thicker and softer because of increased oil secretions from the sebaceous glands. As the skin plumps up, your wrinkles diminish, giving you a somewhat younger appearance.

Bladder/Pelvic Floor

Sex hormones also maintain the firm tone of the pelvic muscles. When estrogen dwindles, muscle tone diminishes and the uterus, bladder, and vagina can drop to varying degrees. This condition is called *prolapse.* If the bladder descends, it is called a *cystocele.* When the rectum prolapses into the vagina, it is called a *rectocele.* (These conditions are illustrated in figure 4 in chapter 3.)

Symptoms of prolapse are usually described as a "feeling of something coming down" or as "a sense of heaviness." If the bladder is involved, coughing, sneezing, or laughing may cause a little urine to leak out despite your best intentions not to permit it. This situation is called *stress incontinence.* There are four successful treatments available for these problems:

1. Pelvic exercises help mild cases only, but should be tried. They simply involve contracting or tightening the pelvic muscles as often as you can, but no fewer than ten times a day. One woman we know does her pelvic floor exercises every time she is waiting at a red light, whether walking or driving. Another does ten pelvic contractions each time she answers the telephone. Attaching this exercise to another daily activity makes it easier to remember to do.
2. Estrogens can improve the muscle tone of the pelvic floor and are of value in mild cases.
3. Pessaries and rings are plastic devices inserted by the gynecologist to lift up the organs. They are used to delay surgery, or if the patient cannot for some reason undergo an operation.
4. Surgical repair is the best treatment. Because prolapse is not a disease, surgery should be considered only if you have troublesome symptoms. Young women who still wish to enlarge their families can have the repair operation in which the uterus, in addition to the ovaries, is left intact. Otherwise, the most effective results are obtained if the uterus is removed, an operation called vaginal hysterectomy with repair.

Remember that the most important function of the vagina is to enable you to enjoy an active and fulfilling sex life. Women who think that their vaginas are stretched and no longer permit them favorable sexual sensation can consider vaginal repair operations. These will tighten the pelvic muscles and narrow the vagina. No woman should be embarrassed to discuss this problem and its repair with her doctor. Sexual pleasure represents a vital aspect of life.

Before thinking of vaginal repair surgery, you should know that bladder symptoms frequently regress when you start to take HRT. Urge incontinence, a disruptive symptom that causes a severe urge to empty the bladder even when it contains very little urine, is frequently eliminated by HRT.

Breast Firmness

Many women feel changes in their breasts during their normal monthly cycle. These changes are a result of the changing levels of their sex hormones. Loss of hormones can result in smaller breasts in slim women. Estrogen treatment may be of value in restoring firmness to breasts. All patients and especially those with fibrocystic breast disease should have regular breast checkups and mammography, when indicated. However, estrogen should not be used as a treatment to develop the breasts.

Longer Life

You know that cardiovascular disease and osteoporosis, two major causes of death, can be reduced or delayed by the appropriate use of HRT. A study conducted between 1971 and 1976 by ten North American Lipid Research Clinics shows that estrogen use can save lives. It reduces mortality from heart disease by one-third. Thus, a woman on estrogen can anticipate more than a four-year increase in her life expectancy.

So, You Decide

The risks and benefits of HRT have been fully explained. You need to consider them individually. Some women, for medical reasons, cannot even consider taking estrogens. They should consider following the other aspects of the Utian Program carefully. Others may have strong and compelling reasons that call for the immediate use of HRT.

Whatever your individual situation, it is of crucial importance that you discuss these matters with your physician. With all factors taken into account, the potential risks of HRT can be minimized by appropriate screening, physician follow-up, and special tests. Moreover, taking the correct hormones in the correct dose in the correct therapy regimen can maximize their benefits.

In our minds, for those women without strict contraindications, there appears to be little doubt that the potential value of HRT outweighs its potential risks. It is the minimax concept. If you can and do choose to take HRT, the responsibility rests with you to consult your doctor at regular intervals. It is up to your physician to supervise your therapy. Let's look at the choice one of my patients made.

The Story of Sallie

Sallie is a sixty-four-year-old attorney. A partner in a large corporate law firm, she is a trial lawyer with a clear, sharp mind. She is married to Richard, has three married children, six grandchildren, and a good housekeeper. All of that was not easy to get or to keep.

At the age of forty-seven, after a few years of menstrual oddities and minor discomforts to which she paid very little attention, Sallie experienced natural menopause. Her periods stopped. After a few months of hot flashes and slight discomfort with intercourse, her physician suggested that she take conjugated estrogen, dosage 1.25 milligrams. Within weeks she began to feel like her old self.

Then, in 1975, a cancer scare was launched by medical reports indicating that estrogen caused uterine cancer. Like women everywhere, Sallie reluctantly gave up her "wonder drug." Her hot flashes resumed, her vaginal lining began to thin again, and sexual intercourse became a painful chore. She became depressed, and she no longer slept well.

There was not much her doctor could do to help, so he gave her tranquilizers to improve her sleep, which eroded what had remained of her sex life. For the next five years, Sallie accepted the changes in her body and in her marriage. She worked harder than ever, because her mind didn't seem to work as quickly anymore.

In 1980, new data showed a new way to prescribe estrogen, along with progestin. The medical reports had shown that this type of cycling lessened the cancer risk greatly. It was at this time that Sallie consulted me, describing herself as "deteriorating," and her life as becoming "less interesting."

We discussed the risk/benefit ratio of estrogen and progestin therapy and I told her to consider all of the facts, decide what she wanted to do, and come back and tell me. She laughed and said, "Bring back my periods. I can't go on this way." I prescribed estrogen in a 0.625-milligram dose and cycled it with 5 milligrams of progestin. Six weeks later, she called me to tell me she was "feeling great!"

In 1985, I established a complete menopause clinic in Cleveland, Ohio, where exercise evaluation, mammography, bone density testing, and diet counseling were done in addition to routine examinations and tests. More and more women who came to us learned of ways to improve their lives, their minds, and their bodies. It seemed as if medicine for women had come of age at last.

Then, on August 3, 1989, the other shoe dropped. The prestigious *New England Journal of Medicine* published a report from Sweden questioning whether HRT with estrogen and progestin doubled the risk of breast cancer. Sallie and hundreds of other frantic women called my office to find out what to do. One by one, I discussed the risks and the benefits based on each woman's individual medical history. I suggested that each woman choose for herself, realizing the risks.

Sallie is still in practice. At age sixty-four, she is still "feeling great." She chose to stay on HRT because she could not even envision facing the deleterious effects of menopause again. She assured me that she understood the medical predicament caused by this new information and promised to be faithful in keeping her future appointments. She will come in every six months for her medical evaluation, confident that she is doing all that she can to pursue her treatment safely. She weighed her risk/benefit ratio and made the decision that was best for her.

·7·

The Utian Menopause Dietstyle: Eating Right for Life

The Utian Menopause Dietstyle encourages you to use your diet as a form of preventive medicine, helping you to feel good and enjoy the rest of your life.

Facts about Midlife Metabolism

"You are what you eat" is never more true than at midlife when your metabolism slows down. At this age for many women, a period of dietary indiscretion or eating unwisely while on a vacation or during a time of stress can play havoc emotionally and physically. In other words, your midlife metabolism does not permit much fooling yourself with food.

Beginning in your mid-thirties, and compounded by menopause, which usually begins in your early fifties, your food intake needs to be scaled back to accommodate your slower metabolism. Nature has rigged our basal metabolic rate (BMR) to slow down after the age of twenty-five, sliding between one-half and one percent per year. It happens gradually, so that it may be some time before you realize that you can't eat the way you once did. If you continue to consume the same amounts and kinds of food that you have in the past, you will have difficulty keeping your figure.

This is the age when even those women who have not had to do so previously may begin each day with a new ritual: praying to the bathroom scale. They get on the scale gently to keep the pointer from going up too quickly or jiggling too much. Finally, they look at the dial on the scale knowing well that whatever the scale reveals will dictate their level of self-satisfaction for the day. "I've lost weight" equals "I like me."

"Therefore, today I'll dress nicely and I'll look terrific. I'll eat less and exercise more, and everything will go well with me today!"

Conversely, "I've gained weight" means "I've been bad." A woman berates herself: "I'm so disgusted with me. No matter what I do, I can't lose weight. I might as well eat whatever I like because I won't look good today anyway." Or it may mean, "I'll try harder today to diet and exercise, but I'm still unhappy with myself."

These feelings can influence the quality of a woman's interpersonal contacts that day as well as her dietary behavior. They may even influence her interest in sex. Although the problems of being over-weight and having a poor diet affect high blood pressure, cholesterol, diabetes, and a host of other diseases and conditions, we also know that for many women diet is an important social and emotional issue.

Facts about Food and Lifestyles

Matching your nutrition habits to your healthy midlife lifestyle is what this chapter is all about. It is also about personal characteristics like self-control and taking pleasure in setting and meeting long-term goals rather than seeking immediate gratification. Most important, it is about caring for and about yourself.

Eating is social; it's pleasurable; it's soothing. All cultures use food to celebrate the special occasions of life. Food, in our society, is less synonymous with our body's survival than it is with the concepts of celebration and reward.

At midlife, you should be seeking a balanced life and beginning a lifestyle that will enhance and ensure your good health. You are looking forward to living longer and living better. Therefore, it becomes necessary to create a balance between overindulgence in food and quasistarvation, and to create within this balance room for the celebrations of life. It is time to replace both the Rubenesque image of the too well-rounded female of the seventeenth century and Tom Wolfe's image of the "social x-rays" of the late twentieth century. In order to foster long-term health, a dietstyle has to be practical and useful.

The Utian Menopause Dietstyle means the end of yo-yo dieting, in which you can't win for losing. With each upswing of the diet yo-yo your body becomes comprised of more fat and less muscle. It is a metabolic fact, proven time and time again. Here's how your metabolism sabotages you. Let's say you go on a strict diet and you lose twenty pounds quickly. Of the twenty pounds you've lost, fifteen pounds were fat and five were muscle. Once off the highly restrictive diet, you regain the weight, faster than the last time because your body has slowed down its metabolism in order to make the most of the very few calories you have been allowing it. It cannot handle the sudden increase in postdiet calories. Now *that* twenty pounds regained is comprised of about eighteen pounds of fat and two pounds of muscle. Each time you yo-yo you become fatter. It's a no-win, or perhaps we should say, a no-lose weight situation.

To make matters worse, medical research has demonstrated that as a woman ages, her percentage of body fat goes up and the percentage of lean body mass or muscle tends to go down. Women often decline in size following menopause. It is lean body mass or muscle mass that is shrinking. As much as 10 percent to 20 percent can be lost through the aging process alone. This percentage increases substantially for the longtime yo-yo dieter. Statistics show that a decrease in size plus a decrease in exercise requires a substantial decrease in the number of calories you eat as you get older, if you want to keep from gaining weight. You must exercise to keep and build lean muscle mass and to fight the body's natural desire to store fat.

Benefits of the Utian Menopause Dietstyle

When you incorporate the Utian Menopause Dietstyle into your life, your entire being benefits. It is not a quick weight-loss diet. It is a wonderful beginning with no end in sight. It makes allowances for mistakes and transgressions, and it enables you to celebrate with a gourmet meal on occasion knowing that you can face yourself, your family, your friends, and your scale without having to face the music tomorrow!

Studies are just beginning to show that better nutrition, increased weight-bearing exercise, and HRT that is appropriate for you may work to arrest the decline in bone mass that puts women at risk of osteoporosis in midlife and later. Such studies also show the benefits of supplemental calcium in the diet. Earlier we believed that bone loss was permanent, but new studies point toward a more hopeful path for women with osteoporosis. Thus, as women grow older, the balance between the various food groups—carbohydrates, proteins, and fats—the types of calories eaten, and the nature and amount of exercise to offset calorie intake become increasingly important. Calories are energy, and regular exercise doesn't just burn more calories when you are doing it; it also gears your body to burn more calories for hours afterward. We will explain this phenomenon in chapter 8.

Appropriate nutrition is a natural pathway toward healthy bone. Bone requires a healthy foundation of protein, in which minerals—especially calcium—are deposited. Successful bone-building requires a diet of well-balanced foods containing adequate calcium.

If you are premenopausal, you need at least 1,000 milligrams of calcium per day. After menopause, your need rises to 1,400 milligrams daily. The average woman in the United States between the ages of forty-five and sixty-five receives far too little calcium: between 460 and 650 milligrams per day. You need to double that amount.

Research is underway to study whether increasing calcium intake during the formative adolescent and young adult years will increase the amount of bone in the later reproductive years. The facts are not in, but it appears that there are no disadvantages to trying that approach.

There have been no studies that prove that a decrease in osteoporosis-related bone fractures can result from dietary changes alone. Nor can calcium supplements alone reduce the incidence of fractures. Making new bone requires the presence of estrogen in your system. This process is enhanced by adequate weight-bearing exercise *and* a good diet that provides the right amount of calcium. Diet and exercise alone will not prevent bone loss!

Determining Your Menopause Dietstyle

When you follow the Utian Menopause Dietstyle program you are taking responsibility for your own body and body image. Once you determine your Utian Dietstyle Program, learn the total number of calories you can consume, and select the number of calories you will expend through exercise—you can then forget about counting calories! It's easy, and the information on pages 106 to 113 tells you how. We will teach you how to customize your dietstyle through appropriate food allowances and exchanges. Once you start doing this repeatedly, you will soon be able to judge portion size by sight. The ability to "judge" a portion will become second nature: Half orders and shared orders will become an integral part of your home and restaurant dining. Of course, no one should begin any dietstyle or exercise program without consulting her physician.

Before you can individualize your dietstyle, it is important to know where in the Utian Menopause Dietstyle you should begin. So, it's time to categorize yourself. Be honest. Using your current weight and your current exercise program, put yourself in one of the three categories listed below.

Average/Active

Are you of average body weight and an active exerciser? Find out by checking your weight range prescribed by your height and body build in the weight chart located at the back of the book in appendix C.

Is your minimum output of exercise at least thirty minutes, four times per week, at 60 percent to no more than 75 percent of your maximum heart rate? (That rate is calculated by subtracting your age from 220 and taking 60 to 75 percent of that number.) Thus, if you are fifty years old, you do the following equation:

$$
\begin{array}{r}
220 \\
\underline{-50} \text{ (your age)} \\
170 \text{ (your maximum heart rate)}
\end{array}
$$

Now, take 60 percent of 170 and you learn that 102 is the lowest number of heart beats per minute that you should aim for when doing aerobic exercise. Take 75 percent, which is 128, and never exceed that number. Calculate your rate now. If, after doing your calculations, your answer to both these questions is yes, you fit comfortably into the Average/Active Dietstyle category and you can consume up to 2,000 of the *right* calories per day to maintain your current weight. There is much more about exercise in chapter 8, in which you will be shown how to put this equation to work for you.

Average/Occasional

This dietstyle category offers up to 1,600 calories per day to women who are of average body weight according to the tables in appendix C, but who are only occasional exercisers. The exercise range chart in chapter 8 points out the range of activity of the occasional exerciser.

A woman falls into this category if she does not exercise three to four times per week for at least thirty minutes at 70 to 80 percent of her maximum heart rate on a regular basis. Here, the operative word is *regular.* If you are this woman, the consumption of 1,600 calories per day should maintain your average body weight. A change in your exercise pattern from occasional to active will create significant weight loss.

Overweight/Nonexerciser

This category is for women who are 25 percent above their average, or ideal, body weight as determined by the table in appendix C. This dietstyle will enable you to achieve significant weight loss. It is important to understand the unalterable fact that 3,500 calories constitute one pound of body weight. Therefore, in order to lose one pound of body fat per week, you must consume 3,500 fewer calories per week. The most you should ever try to lose per week for a healthful and long-term effect is two pounds, which means eliminating 7,000 calories per week through diet or burning more calories through increased exercise. Once you fully understand the expenditure of calories through exercise, you can understand the whole secret of weight loss. No magic, just mathematics! As a woman in this category of the Utian Dietstyle, you will need to drop your calorie intake to 1,000 calories per day and add exercise to your daily routine. If you are more than 40 percent over your desired body weight, for faster weight loss you can drop to the 800-calorie-per-day dietstyle and add regular exercise to your program until you reach your appropriate weight according to the table in appendix C. Then return to the 1,000-calorie dietstyle. You should never consider eating fewer than 800 calories per day, and these calories need to be carefully balanced between the six basic food groups.

What's in the Dietstyle for You?

The rest of this chapter will provide you with the complete details of the Utian Menopause Dietstyle, along with suggested menus; easy ways to evaluate the nutritional value of foods; tips for handling portion control, food exchanges, and free calories; and suggestions for changing your attitudes and behaviors toward food.

A Word about Food Exchanges

Food exchanges are a way of looking at the complete value of a portion of food, understanding how and why it is required in your diet, and knowing how to replace or exchange it for another food, without changing the nutrient and caloric value. For example, one fruit does not necessarily exchange evenly for another, but might get you more pieces or only a portion of another. One small apple does not exchange for one apricot; it gets you three. But, ten cherries can be swapped for only one-half grapefruit—no more, no less. Better yet, you can trade one-half bagel or one-half English muffin for a whole slice of bread. Food exchanges are an important aspect of our dietstyle, because they enable you to eliminate boredom in your diet without sabotaging your good intentions. Complete lists of food exchanges for each category follow the three dietstyle menus.

The 2,000-Calorie Dietstyle for the Average/Active Woman

Daily Menu

Use foods from the food exchange lists (pages 110–113) in each food category. They offer you the variety and the ability to create a wide variety of meals within these general guidelines.

Breakfast
    2 Fruits
    2 Eggs, poached or boiled (once a week only)
    Fish (6-ounce portion)
    1 Tomato (if desired)
    2 Starches (preferably unsweetened cereal)
    Orange juice (unsweetened, 4 ounces)
    Regular or decaffeinated coffee or tea, limit 2 cups (If milk is
        used it must come from daily allowance.)

Midmorning Snack
    Herb tea or decaffeinated coffee (with milk from daily
        allowance)

Lunch
   2 Average portions of lean meat (6 ounces/150 grams); or
      poultry, skin removed (6 ounces/150 grams); or fish (8
      ounces/240 grams); or skimmed-milk cheese (4 ounces/100
      grams)
   Vegetables, cooked or raw, or in salads (unlimited)
   2 Starches
   2 Fruits
   Herb tea or decaffeinated coffee (with milk from daily
      allowance)

Midafternoon Snack
   Herb tea or decaffeinated coffee (with milk from daily
      allowance)
   Any vegetable listed (if desired)

Dinner
   Lean meat, skinless poultry, fish, or skimmed-milk cheese
      (6–8-ounce portion)
   Unlimited vegetables and salad
   2 Starches
   2 Fruits
   Herb tea or decaffeinated coffee (with milk from daily
      allowance)

Other Daily Allowances
   Low-fat milk (16 ounces)
   Margarine (2 level teaspoons)
   Reduced-calorie salad dressing (1 tablespoon)
   Diet soda and mineral waters (unlimited)—limit high-sodium
      drinks to one a day
   Clear soups, meat and vegetable extracts (as desired)
   Vinegar, pepper, herbs, and spices (as desired)

Important Notes. Avoid sugar; do not add any to coffee or tea. Use
artificial sweetener, as desired. Foods should be boiled, baked,
stewed, steamed, microwaved, poached, or grilled without fat. Do not
fry foods or sauté them in fat. Try to be aware of the salt content in
food by carefully reading the labels on processed foods. It is not
always easy to tell where salt is hidden.

The 1,600-Calorie Dietstyle for the Average/Occasional Woman

Daily Menu
Selecting foods from the food exchange lists (pages 110–113) in each food category offers you the variety and the ability to create you own meals within these broad general guidelines.

Breakfast
  2 Fruits
  1 Egg, boiled or poached (twice a week only) or fish (3-ounce portion)
  Tomato, if desired
  2 Starches
  Herb tea or coffee, or decaffeinated coffee (with milk from daily allowance)

Midmorning Snack
  Herb tea or decaffeinated coffee (milk from daily allowance)

Lunch
  Lean meat (up to 4 ounces); or skinless poultry (4 ounces); or fish (5 ounces); or skimmed-milk cheese (3 ounces)
  Vegetables and salads from vegetable list, unlimited
  2 Starches
  1 Fruit
  Herb tea or decaffeinated coffee (with milk from daily allowance)

Midafternoon Snack
  Herb tea or decaffeinated coffee (milk from daily allowance)
  Any vegetable listed (if desired)

Dinner
  Lean meat, poultry, fish, or skimmed-milk cheese (6-ounce portion)
  Vegetables and salad, unlimited
  1 Starch
  1 Fruit
  Herb tea or decaffeinated coffee (with milk from daily allowance)

The Other Daily Allowances and Notes from the 2,000-calorie diet apply to all other dietstyles.

The 1,000-Calorie Dietstyle for the Overweight/Nonexerciser

Daily Menu
This basic diet can be followed safely by women in all three groups, but it is essential for women more than 25 percent over their ideal weight who do not exercise. As with the other dietstyles, select foods from the exchange lists (pages 110–113) in each food category. These offer as much variety as possible.

Breakfast
  1 Fruit
  1 Egg, poached or boiled (twice a week only), or 3 ounces of
    fish
  Tomato, if desired
  1 Starch
  Coffee, decaffeinated or regular, or tea with milk from daily
    allowance (if desired)—you may have up to 2 cups of
    caffeinated coffee for breakfast

Midmorning Snack
  Herb tea or decaffeinated coffee (with milk from daily
    allowance)

Lunch
  Lean meat (3 ounces); or poultry (3 ounces); or fish (4 ounces);
    or skimmed-milk cheese (2 ounces)
  Vegetables or salads
  1 Starch
  1 Fruit
  Herb tea or decaffeinated coffee (with milk from daily
    allowance)

Midafternoon Snack
  Herb tea or decaffeinated coffee (with milk from daily
    allowance)
  Any vegetables listed (if desired)

Dinner
  Lean meat, poultry, fish, or skimmed-milk cheese (3–4-ounce
    portion)
  Unlimited vegetables and salad
  1 Starch
  1 Fruit
  Herb tea or decaffeinated coffee (with milk from daily
    allowance)

The Other Daily Allowances and Notes from the 2,000-calorie dietstyle apply to all other dietstyles.

Special Guidelines for the 800-Calorie Dietstyle

If you want to follow the 800-calorie dietstyle, consult with your
doctor and find out if it is safe for you and for how long you can
remain on the 800-calorie dietstyle. If you get a medical okay, go
ahead with this dietstyle—it's easy to follow. Just omit two starch
exchanges and one fruit exchange from the 1,000-calorie dietstyle.
Watch your selections carefully, so that you eat enough calcium-rich
foods. The list of calcium-rich foods is in appendix B.

Food Exchange Lists That Apply to All Dietstyles

Vegetable Exchanges
Eat as much as you like of the following vegetables:

artichoke (leaves)	asparagus	beet greens
bean sprouts	broccoli	brussel sprouts
cabbage	carrots	cauliflower
celery	chard	Chinese cabbage
collard greens	cucumber	eggplant
endive	escarole	green peppers
Jerusalem artichokes	jicama	lettuce
kale	leeks	onion
mushrooms	okra	peppers
parsley	pea pods, Chinese	rutabagas
pimentos	radishes	squash
sauerkraut	shallots	string beans

scallions	spinach	turnip greens
summer squash	tomato	watercress
turnips	water chestnuts	

Carbohydrate Exchanges (Starches)

The following foods are interchangeable portion for portion. Each amount listed represents one portion of starch:

- 1 thin slice of bread (equals 1 ounce)
- 2 medium-size potatoes
- 2 tablespoons rice, macaroni, spaghetti, or other pasta noodles
- 3 tablespoons beans, peas, or sweet potatoes
- 3 tablespoons cereal
- 3 crackers
- 2 tablespoons reduced-calorie ice cream
- 2 teaspoons cocoa
- 1 tablespoon nuts

Fruit Exchanges

Any of the following fruits are interchangeable. Each amount represents one portion. Fruit may be eaten raw, stewed, or baked:

1 small apple	⅓ cup apple juice	⅓ cup applesauce
3 small apricots	½ small banana	½ cup berries
½ cantaloupe	10 cherries	1 small fig
½ grapefruit	½ cup grapefruit juice	12 grapes
½ cup honeydew melon	1 small orange	½ cup orange juice
1 medium peach	1 small pear	½ cup pineapple
½ cup pineapple juice	2 plums	6 prunes
1 cup strawberries	1 tangerine	1 large slice watermelon
½ cup fresh fruit salad (made of any assortment of fruits)		

A Word about Water

Water may be your best ally in your war against weight. It is a natural appetite suppressor and it helps your body to metabolize stored fat.

It is a natural diuretic, so you can get rid of excess water, or edema. Water helps to maintain good muscle tone and helps your body rid itself of waste. No matter which dietstyle you follow, you should drink eight 8-ounce glasses of water every day.

Foods to Avoid or Omit

Omit the following foods from your daily dietstyle except for on rare occasions: sugar, glucose, jams, honey, syrup, candy, chocolate, cakes, sweet biscuits, pastries, puddings, cookies, sweetened canned fruits, some oils, fats, sausages, bacon, fried foods, beer, sweet wines, and alcohol.

Be careful with the following cholesterol-rich foods (use only the amounts allowed in your dietstyle): butter, cheese (low-fat or skimmed-milk cheeses), eggs, lard, red meat (eat once a week only), and anything made with saturated fats. Please refer to the tables relating to calcium, cholesterol, and fat in your diet. They appear in appendix B.

Special Celebrations and the Free Calorie System

On special occasions you need to know how to eat, so that you do not feel that you have unalterably ruined your new dietstyle and become so discouraged that you quit taking care of yourself nutritionally. When you work with a daily dietstyle calorie number and use our system of food exchanges, it is only a matter of mathematics and planning. Consider that twice a week you can go to a party, dinner, or any other special event where food is featured and use our "free calories" system to guide you.

By "free," we mean you choose among several options. On your two special-occasion days, raise your caloric intake by 500 calories. Thus, if you are on the 1,000-calorie dietstyle, on those two occasions you can consume 1,500 calories, which gives you 500 free calories at each event—enough to have a cocktail, a glass of wine, a dessert, or something else that you especially miss and want. But you must balance your account by *deleting* those extra 1,000 calories during the rest of the week. How? It's easy. Just go on the 800-calorie dietstyle for the other five days.

This 500-calorie, twice-a-week increase for special occasions applies to all of the dietstyles. However, no more than 500 extra calories should be consumed at any one time and they should always be paid back within the same week. If you choose your portion exchanges appropriately, and use your free calories wisely, you can go out and celebrate without feeling deprived or derelict in your dietary duties to yourself.

Twenty-four Tips for Transforming Your Attitudes and Behaviors Toward Food

Now that you are working toward a longer and healthier life, it is important to begin to understand how old habits work against your new dietstyle. The following is a list of ideas for modifying your behavior to support your healthy eating habits. Because behavior modification is a gradual process, select from the following list seven changes that you'd like to make and add two more only when you feel that you have incorporated the first seven into your dietstyle. Then, add two more, and two more, and so on until you have changed how you eat and your new dietstyle is working easily for you.

1. Keep focused on the present as you work toward your future good health. Congratulate yourself for whatever steps you took today in achieving your goals.
2. Set realistic goals for making positive changes in your life.
3. Never go grocery shopping when you are hungry.
4. Shop with a list and follow that list.
5. Shop with the approximate amount of money you will need to buy only the items on your list.
6. Go directly to what you need to purchase; don't browse for other ideas for food.
7. Plan, whenever possible, to schedule your meals around your personal hungry times.
8. Plan what you will eat and eat only what you planned.
9. Try to eat your meals in the same location at home.
10. Never stand, eat, and run.
11. Do not eat out of containers. Plan your portion and fix a plate for yourself.
12. Use smaller plates and bowls so that they appear fuller to you.
13. Learn how to say no to foods that you are being pressured to eat. If "no" is not working try the following:

- "I'm too full."
- "I'm allergic."
- "My doctor doesn't permit me to eat this."
- "Thanks, it was delicious, and exactly enough for me."

14. Do not confuse tiredness with hunger; if you are tired, try to lie down and sleep or rest.
15. Do not confuse boredom with hunger; if bored, call an interesting friend or read a good book.
16. Stay out of the kitchen whenever possible.
17. Try to stay away from "eating friends": those whom you only meet to eat with.
18. When eating out, eat a portion of free vegetable first so you are less hungry. A large salad helps a lot.
19. When you get the urge to eat at a party, start a conversation instead.
20. At a restaurant, order dishes that take a long time to eat: paella, bouillabaisse, cioppino, Chinese food, Japanese food, or any other foods that you can eat with chopsticks.
21. Give up elastic and expandable waistlines. When your clothes are tight, feel it, and know it.
22. If you are trying to reduce, imagine how good you will feel; visualize how good you will look.
23. If you are maintaining your dietstyle, think about what caring for yourself means to you now and in the future.
24. Be decisive and focused about your intention to eat the way that makes you feel great! Let no obstacles steer you away from your course. The Utian Menopause Dietstyles are designed to reeducate your appetite, to help you be selective about what you eat, and to gradually modify your behavior toward foods. This dietstyle, coupled with a regular exercise program as described in chapter 8, should help you to feel confident that you are doing your part to claim a longer and healthier life.

How to Begin Your Dietstyle

1. Make up your mind that you will take complete control of and responsibility for what you eat and for how you look.
2. Review the dietstyle categories to determine where you fit.

3. Make a contract with yourself:
   I will begin the _____ calorie dietstyle on _____,
   19_____. My current weight is _____; my goal weight, according to the table in appendix C, is _____ pounds.
4. If necessary, remove from your kitchen those foods that are irresistible to you.
5. Make a shopping list using your dietstyle menu and the exchange lists.
6. Fill in the following sentence that describes your present mood:
   When I made the decision to incorporate my dietstyle into my life, I made a commitment to *me*. I was feeling

   _____

   _____

   _____ when I made that choice.
7. Review this section, particularly point 6, whenever you feel that you are slipping in your resolve.

A Week's Worth of Dietstyle Planning

Until the process of exchanging foods for one another becomes second nature to you, plan your weekly menu in advance, building into it those special-occasion free calories. The following sample chart can be easily duplicated on a copying machine or written in a notebook and kept close at hand:

MY DIETSTYLE PLANNING AND FOOD EXCHANGE GRAPH
Utian Menopause Management Program

Dietstyle _____ Week _____ Date _____ Weight _____

	Monday	Tuesday	Wednesday	Thursday	Friday	Saturday	Sunday
Exchange/Occasion/Calories							
Breakfast							
Mid. A.M.							
Lunch							
Mid P.M.							
Dinner							

During week number _____, I was completely successful _____
moderately successful _____
marginally successful _____
unsuccessful _____

Plan week _____. Keep up the good work or try even harder.

·8·

Getting Physical:
Exercise and Sports

Move it or lose it is the key to keeping your body strong and flexible, but it is never more true than for women at menopause. Women are jogging and jumping, twisting and turning, swimming and cycling as never before as they realize the benefits of exercise. There are so many choices: walking, running, swimming, weight lifting, bicycling, rowing, plus a vast array of racquet sports, competitive team games such as volleyball, the martial arts, and all kinds of dance. It's your choice. To secure your continued good health and independence later in life, it is important that you do choose and that you do exercise! In this chapter, we'll give you a rundown of the types of exercise we recommend as aerobic and weight-bearing activities plus our own specially designed exercises for strengthening muscles and conserving bone mass.

Exercise Fights Osteoporosis

Weight-bearing exercise is a natural approach to the prevention of osteoporosis. We explained earlier that you can prevent osteoporosis if you take control of two main factors. First, you need to develop as much bone as possible during the formative years, before menopause. Second, you have to reduce the rate of bone loss that may occur after menopause.

In order to reduce bone loss, you must make certain lifestyle changes. Many studies have shown conclusively that an inappropriate diet, lack of exercise, and smoking can result in loss of bone. We have already discussed diet and smoking; this chapter gives you the exercises you need to do to meet your goal.

What You Can Expect from Exercise

Exercise may enhance bone mass and bone density. To see a good example, compare the arms of your favorite tennis player. You will find that the dominant arm is larger; it has developed more bone and muscle from use. Then think of the astronauts traveling through space with little opportunity to exercise against any resistance in the weightlessness of space. They lose bone.

Moderate exercise is very beneficial; excess exercise may not be. Let's look at one more extreme example. Take a woman who is following an overly strenuous exercise program. Let's say she is a marathon runner. She may lose her menstrual period, because through excessive exercise she has altered ovarian activity and reduced her body fat so much that her body's production of estrogen is inhibited. She will then lose bone, as well.

Exercise offers emotional benefit as well as physical energy by altering your state of mood. This alteration probably occurs because exercise activates the release of certain hormones within the brain that we call the *central endorphins* or, *brain morphines.* They produce that special sense of well-being that we experience after exercise.

Recent studies directed specifically toward menopausal women have shown that vigorous exercise reduces muscle tension and decreases anxiety significantly. The relief of anxiety is often the result of an increase in the levels of epinephrine and *norepinephrine* circulating in your blood. These substances improve *neurotransmission,* or *nerve messages.* Similar studies have proved that the nature of sleep improves for exercisers and the physically fit.

As we said earlier, a problem with exercise is poor compliance. Women start an exercise program, lose interest, and drop out usually sometime during the first three months of a program. Most studies show that the mood-enhancing results of regular exercise only develop strongly after three months, coinciding with when you arrive at a state of physical fitness. Other studies also suggest that good physical exercise, continued late into life, will reduce the aging of your brain and offer you more vigor and consistency of performance into very late old age.

Choosing an exercise activity that is fun for you is as important as getting active, because if it's not fun you won't stick with it. Also select a variety of activities, so you are less bored while you enhance your flexibility, strength, and endurance. We know that more women have gotten more active since the 1960s, but we also know that not enough women exercise. Exercise benefits every system in your body, which is probably why it makes you feel so good. There is also a special look to the physically fit woman: a look of strength, confidence, and glowing good health. Her step is lighter, her handshake firmer, and her gaze clearer. These are not appearances without foundation; they are a direct result of the flexibility, strength, and better oxygenation of the body that a regular and well-defined exercise program begets.

Today's models and movie stars alike aim for healthy bodies that appear strong and sturdy. A woman with well-built shoulders no longer conveys a masculine image, but rather that of a woman who looks like she can take care of herself. With more women than ever before in the rough-and-tumble work force, and with women living longer than ever before, exercise becomes the path to a very important degree of strength and self-sufficiency.

Note: It is vitally important before you begin an exercise program to have a complete medical checkup to assure that the program you are about to begin is right for you. Let's review the broad range of benefits that exercise offers women at midlife and how it may offset some of the problems that hormonal changes can cause.

Many physicians suggest exercise as a treatment for depression. Studies show that exercise aids sleep and can overcome a general feeling of nervousness, both complaints of postmenopausal women. Certain kinds of exercises strengthen bone and aid flexibility so that we do not get hurt as often, or as badly, and we heal faster, too. We know that exercise causes the reproductive system to work better, but that it must be pursued wisely, since perimenopausal women who jog or run excessively can lose their periods entirely and, as a result, lose the bone-building benefits of estrogen.

Goals of the Right Exercise Program

As our bodies age, we can lose aerobic capacity, flexibility, and strength. Studies have shown that calcium and vitamin D are necessary for healthy bone growth, but must be combined with exercise to be fully used by the skeletal system. There are appropriate goals for your exercise program that need to be reached through properly selected and executed activities; otherwise your exercise program may not serve your body well and may even be injurious.

Exercise should be incorporated into your lifestyle on a regular basis and should be structured to accomplish these five specific goals.

1. To increase your heart and lung efficiency
2. To increase your muscle strength
3. To increase your muscle tone
4. To increase your muscle endurance
5. To increase your flexibility

Meeting These Exercise Goals

Two kinds of exercise are necessary in order to meet your goals: aerobic exercise and weight-bearing exercise. Aerobic exercise increases your oxygen capacity, because it is a way of exercising that demands extra oxygen. It stimulates beneficial changes in the respiratory and circulatory systems of your body, ultimately making your lungs and your heart work more efficiently, and it is equally important in maintaining your cholesterol and blood lipids at normal levels. Exercise will elevate the HDL cholesterol—the good cholesterol—for most women, and lower the triglycerides. It should also lower the LDL, or bad, cholesterol levels. These changes help cleanse the blood of fats that can block arteries and put you at risk for heart disease.

Aerobic exercise also burns more calories and helps you to reduce body weight and fat. Aerobic exercises include walking, running, jogging, cycling, swimming, cross-country skiing, and dance programs that are designed to use oxygen. The treadmill, the stationary bicycle, the cross-country ski machine, and the stair machine are all capable of helping you get a good aerobic workout when you use them properly, working at 70 to 80 percent of your maximum heart rate for at least twenty minutes, three times a week.

Weight-bearing exercises, those loosely defined as activities that work against gravity, are vital to bone health. Women turn to walking, cycling, golfing, playing tennis, and dancing, to name a few activities that make them lift, push, pull, bend, and stretch. Weight lifting, weight training, and body building also help to save, build, and even rebuild bone. Some studies show that weight-bearing exercises and muscle contractions generate stress on the bone that is necessary to prevent bone loss. Other studies have shown that the decrease in bone density in older women may be halted, or even reversed, when women exercise regularly. Today, women are "pumping iron" as never before, using free weights, barbells, and weight disks, or using weight machines such as Nautilus or Universal at health clubs. (It is important that well-trained instructors teach you how to use the equipment.)

Choosing Your Exercise Plan

If you are ready to make a lifelong commitment to exercise, begin by choosing aerobic activities that are fun for you and combining them with weight-bearing activities that interest you. Try various activities to see which ones get you moving both physically and psychologically. Then, combine various activities and, to keep your level of interest high, vary the combinations.

For example, you may work out a warm-up, aerobic dance routine, and cool-down exercise program that you do three days a week and alternate it with a weight-lifting routine on the intervening days. Or you may walk vigorously three days a week and cycle two days. However you set up your exercise program, vary it when the least bit of boredom creeps in and try new activities or group activities to stimulate your interest.

How Much Should You Exercise?

It depends on whether you have been exercising regularly or are about to begin. Your level of fitness right now and your medical evaluation determine where you begin. When you begin to exercise, or when you begin a new activity, it is important that you start at a low level of participation and build up very slowly. Soreness or injury that sets you back days, weeks, or months is a greater deterrent to achieving fitness than taking it slowly and steadily, gradually increasing the time and the intensity to get to a point of physical fitness sooner. Remember the parable of the tortoise and the hare? Here, too, it is the persevering tortoise that wins.

How Often Should You Exercise?

Plan to exercise four times a week from twenty to forty minutes per session, and try not to slip below three times a week. Remember, you have made a commitment to your own good health and there just has to be time for it. If need be, write your exercise period into your datebook just as you would any other important appointment, and keep it!

Aerobic Exercises

These exercises improve heart and lung activity by forcing the body to use more oxygen. Aerobic fitness can be maintained by participating in an aerobic exercise for twenty minutes or more at least three times per week. The intensity of the activity, once you are in condition for it, should raise your heart rate to between 60 and 75 percent of your maximum heart rate. The table below will enable you to see where you fit in according to your age. The average maximum heart rate has been determined by taking 220 and subtracting your age as we described in chapter 7; your target heart rate is then the appropriate percentage of that rate.

TARGET HEART RATE

Age (Years)	Target Heart Rate (Beats Per Minute)	Average Maximum Heart Rate (Beats Per Minute)
20	120–150	200
25	117–146	195
30	114–142	190
35	111–138	185
40	108–135	180
45	105–131	175
50	102–127	170
55	99–123	165
60	96–120	160
65	93–116	155
70	90–113	150

Source: U.S. Department of Health and Human Services; Public Health Service; National Institutes of Health; National Heart, Lung, and Blood Institute: *Exercise and Your Heart.* NIH Publication No. 81-1677. Washington D.C., U.S. Government Printing Office, 1961.

The following are the three types of aerobic exercises that we recommend, and our suggested goals.

Indoor Stationary Running
Start by standing with your feet together and place your arms at your sides. Begin running with your right leg, raising your foot at least four

inches off the ground. Remember to lift your knees. Count one full step each time your right foot touches the ground.

SUGGESTED GOALS AND DURATION FOR WOMEN AGES 35–65*

Weeks	Steps	Time (Min.)	Ages 35–50 Target		Age 50–65 Target	
1–2	50	4				
3–4	70	4				
5–6	90	4				
7–8	110	4				
9–10	130	4				
11–12	150	4				
13–14	170	5				
15–16	180	5				
17–18	190	5				
19–20	200	5				

Source: Compiled by the author.

*You can time your running period by the clock or you can count the number of times your right foot touches down to arrive at your fixed goal.

Outdoor Walking

Walk briskly, lift your knees, swing your arms, and breathe deeply, but *do not run*. The duration suggested in the table on the next page represents a minimum time.

SUGGESTED GOALS AND DURATION

Weeks	Time
1–2	10 minutes
3–4	12 minutes
5–6	15 minutes
7–thereafter	20 minutes

Source: Compiled by the author.

Swimming

The breast stroke is the recommended style, although the crawl will work, too. Breathe deeply with each full stroke. The following minimum targets are advised.

SUGGESTED GOALS AND DURATION

Weeks	Time	Meters
1–2	3 minutes	at least 50 meters
3–4	5 minutes	at least 75 meters
5–6	7 minutes	at least 100 meters
7–8	9 minutes	at least 150 meters
9–10	10 minutes	150–300 meters

Source: Compiled by the author.

Muscle-Strengthening Exercise

Antiosteoporosis, Back-Strengthening, Body Flexibility Plan
Frequency. At least four times per week.
Number of repetitions. The suggested number of times you
   perform each exercise is included with the description of the
   exercise. For the first two weeks, do only half that number.
   Start slowly, and increase the number of repetitions as you
   feel the benefit of these strengthening exercises.

We have designed eleven exercises specifically for women at midlife, geared toward staving off osteoporosis through strengthening and flexibility. Once you have achieved the maximum number of repetitions, this exercise program should take you less than thirty minutes to complete. It requires so little time for so much benefit! Before beginning it, have a small pillow, a bed pillow, and a straight-back chair nearby. You may find that an exercise mat placed directly on the floor will cushion your body during this series of exercises and make you more comfortable. Dress in comfortable exercise clothing and, if possible, try to do these exercises in front of a mirror so that you can check your positioning. Rhythmic slow music may also add to your enjoyment.

Points to Remember Before You Begin

- Always warm up for at least five minutes before beginning to exercise. Your warm-up routine should use the full range of motion of all your joints.
- Always cool down after exercising. Walking for five minutes is an excellent cool-down.
- All strengthening exercises should be done in a controlled, slow manner. There should be no bouncing or bobbing or rapid jerky movements that may cause injury and do not add to fitness.
- Rest between sets of exercises.
- Practice breathing in a controlled manner during exercise. Do not hold your breath. Do try to exhale during the hardest exertion in an exercise and inhale during the easy part.
- Pain means stop; do not try to work through it.
- The right clothes make the right exercises easier, but the right exercise shoe properly fitted is mandatory. Your athletic shoe store is the place to start. There are shoes that are designed for specific kinds of exercise. Ask your salesperson to explain the advantages of the various designs and materials.

Utian Exercise Program*

The first four exercises are warm-up stretches designed to tone muscles and stimulate bone growth.

*The Bent-Knee switch, Lying back arch, and Knee lift exercises are modified from M. Sinaki, 1982. Postmenopausal spinal osteoporosis: Physical therapy and rehabilitation principles. *Mayo Clin. Proc.* 57:699–703. By permission.

The fifth exercise strengthens the neck and cervical spine.

The sixth exercise strengthens your thighs and your abdominal muscles.

Exercise number seven stretches and strengthens your lower back.

The eighth exercise strengthens your back muscles and stimulates the vertebrae. The eighth and ninth exercises strengthen back and hamstring muscles.

Exercise ten works to strengthen back and abdominal muscles.

The last exercise strengthens thigh muscles and improves deep breathing techniques to enhance heart and lung function.

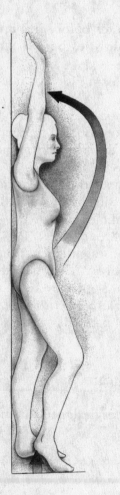

1. *OVERHEAD STRETCH.* Stand with your back straight against a wall. Stretch your right arm as high as possible above your head while you lift your right heel. Keep your back straight against the wall. Hold the stretch for three seconds. Then repeat with the left arm and left heel. Do each side five times.

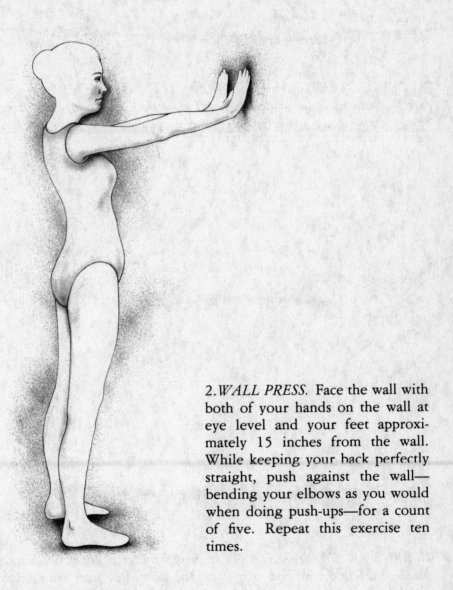

2.*WALL PRESS.* Face the wall with both of your hands on the wall at eye level and your feet approximately 15 inches from the wall. While keeping your back perfectly straight, push against the wall—bending your elbows as you would when doing push-ups—for a count of five. Repeat this exercise ten times.

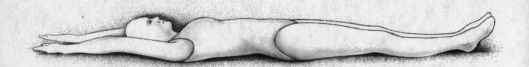

3. *LYING STRETCH.* Lie flat on the floor with your legs and your arms extended as far as possible and your back flat against the floor. Hold each stretch for a count of five. Repeat the stretch ten times.

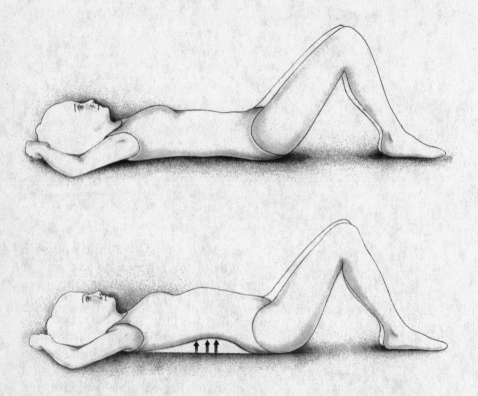

4. *BENT-KNEE FLOOR STRETCH.* Stay flat on the floor. Bend your knees, but keep your feet evenly on the floor. Put your arms above your head, but do not stretch them. Relax. Then tighten the muscles of your buttocks and lower abdomen while flattening your back against the floor. Hold this flattened back position for a count of ten. Relax for a count of three and repeat the exercise ten times.

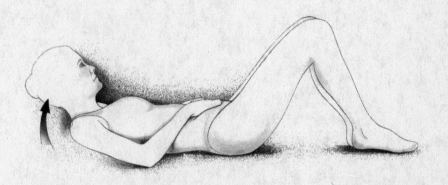

5. *HEAD LIFT.* Still lying on the floor, with your knees bent to approximately a 90-degree angle, put your hands on your abdomen, and with your shoulder in contact with the floor at all times, lift your head a few inches off the floor for a count of five. Then lower your head to the floor. Lift and lower twelve times.

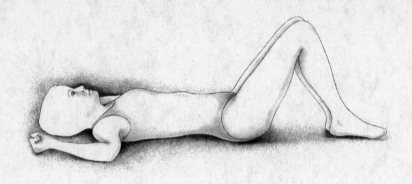

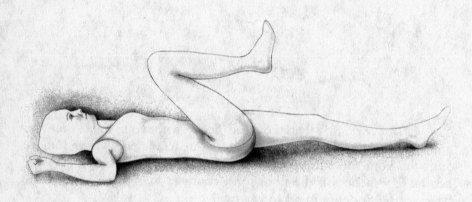

6. *BENT-KNEE SWITCH.* Still on your back, put your arms over your head and bend your knees with both feet flat on the floor. Move one knee toward your chest while straightening the other leg. Return to your original position with both knees bent. Now, switch legs and again relax in your original position. Repeat the exercise using each leg ten times.

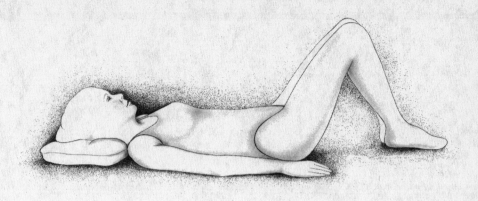

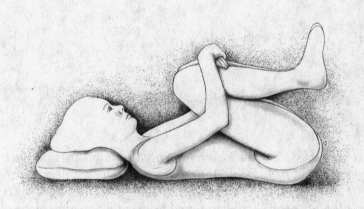

7. *LYING KNEE GRASP.* Don't get up yet. Stay on your back, but this time put a small pillow under your head. Keeping your feet flat on the ground, bend your knees and relax your arms at your sides. Raise your knees to your chest, wrap your hands around your knees, and pull them gently toward your chest, holding them there for a count of ten. During this exercise your shoulders should stay on the mat and your knees should move together. Do a series of three of these exercises, then relax. Repeat until you have completed four sets for a total count of twelve repetitions.

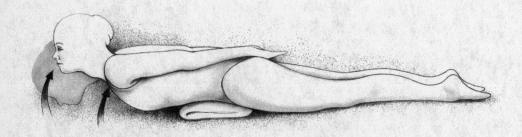

8. *LYING BACK ARCH.* Now roll over on your stomach and place a bed pillow folded in half under your abdomen. Lie face down with arms down beside your body. Lift your arms above the height of your buttocks and lift your head as high as possible, creating an arch in your back, Repeat this exercise twelve times.

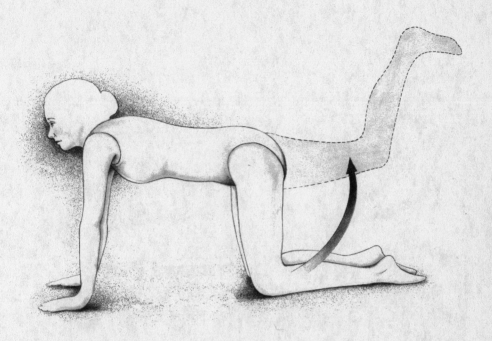

9. *KNEE LIFT.* Come up on your hands and knees. With your elbows locked in position, lift one leg straight back as high as your buttocks, bending your knee to form a straight body line shoulder to knee. Return to starting position and then repeat using the other leg. Do twelve repetitions.

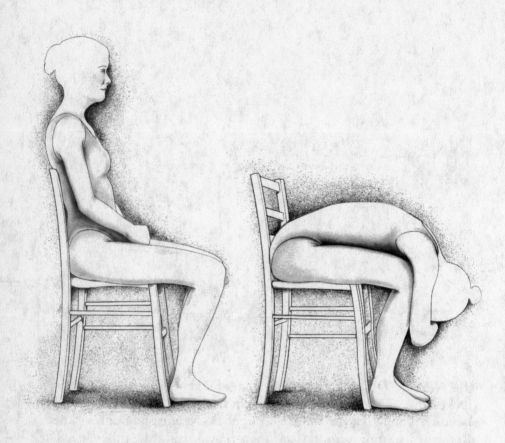

10. *CHAIR SLUMP.* Sit on a straight-back chair and face straight ahead. Fold your arms loosely on your lap. Now drop forward until your head is between your knees and your arms have slid forward toward your ankles. Tighten your abdominal muscles while returning to your starting position. Relax for a count of three and repeat the exercise ten times.

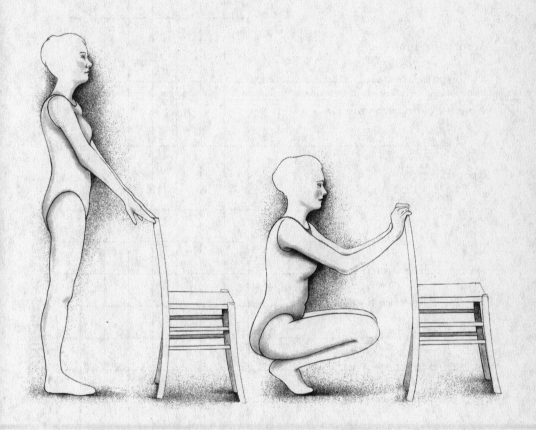

11. *CHAIR SQUAT.* Stand erect while holding onto the back of your chair. Now squat with your back slightly bent. Then stand, relax, and repeat ten times.

If you have not been exercising, is this the day that you will begin? We hope so! In order to help you plan your exercise program, we have developed a chart so that you can monitor your first month's progress. Either make additional copies for yourself on a copying machine or draw a similar chart in your notebook.

My Exercise Regimen

	(Sample)							
Date								
Aerobic Routine								
Type								
Weight-Bearing Routine								
Type								
Utian Program								
1. Overhead stretch								
2. Wall press								
3. Lying stretch								
4. Bent-knee floor stretch								
5. Head lift								
6. Bent-knee switch								
7. Lying knee grasp								
8. Lying back arch								
9. Knee lift								
10. Chair slump								
11. Chair squat								

REPETITIONS OR TIME

·9·

Good, Better, Best:
Sexuality and Aging

Sexuality is not something to overlook just because you are "fiftysomething" or even something much older! Sexuality is a major aspect of all of life. Just as sex is not merely the contact of the genital organs, sexuality goes far deeper than simply your reaction to the levels of sex hormones circulating in your blood. Human sexual awareness is present shortly after birth and, like eating and sleeping, remains a part of our beings until we die. Throughout life, sexuality acts as a source of self-confirmation and as a stimulator and initiator of communication with others. It adds to our drive and determination and fuels our ambition and achievement. Sexuality involves self-understanding, love, intimacy, human contact, caring, friendship, and fun.

Myths, Misconceptions, Stereotypes, and Sexuality

If sexuality has such a broad definition, it must be obvious that it does not mean that you need to be beautiful, youthful, or have a curvaceous figure to enjoy a good sex life. If there is a tragedy concerning sexuality, it is precisely this stereotype. A little research makes it easy to understand how it all began.

In chapter 1, we described how women at midlife were viewed a century ago: "Compelled to yield to the power of time, women now cease to exist as to the species and, henceforward, live only for themselves. Their features are stamped with the impress of age and their genital organs are sealed with the signet of sterility." Such damaging myths spanned the decades to cloud our existence and to perpetuate misunderstanding of the "prime-time" woman. They created and circulated the idea that the male, as he grows older, remains appealing and attractive, whereas the older female becomes asexual. He becomes dignified; she becomes old. Not true!

These misconceptions about sexual function and sexual response after menopause are behind the completely erroneous statements of intelligent people to the effect that, "Sex doesn't matter when you're older," or "An interest in sex is abnormal for older people," or "Remarriage after the death of your spouse should be discouraged." Why?

The climacteric appears to have little effect on sexual functioning. The condition of painful intercourse, called *dyspareunia,* which sometimes occurs, is a complication of the thinning vaginal wall. It does not reflect a loss of libido.

Deeper understanding of the sexuality of the older woman began with the pioneering work of Alfred Kinsey. In his book, *Sexual Behavior in the Human Female,* he reported the results of an extensive survey of sexual behavior in America. Some of the survey questions were designed to elicit degrees of sexual expression. There were middle-aged and older women among those surveyed. For the first time, we learned from their responses that sexuality and sexual response improved after menopause for some of them. Their fears of unwanted pregnancies disappeared along with their periods. The Kinsey report tended to focus purely on genital stimulation and response and to show that women after the age of menopause continued to enjoy sexual gratification. It did not, however, sharply define sexuality.

The issue of sexuality was clarified in the subsequent reports of sex therapists William Masters and Virginia Johnson. Their landmark book, *Human Sexual Response,* was published in 1966. Through their research, and the work of others in the field, we learned that many factors influence sexual behavior. Menopause does not specifically change behavior, nor does aging per se. Of greater importance is your sexuality quotient before menopause, your health, and whether you have an active sexual partner or are divorced, widowed, or living alone.

Determining Your Sexuality

Since sexuality has such a broad definition and is influenced by so many factors—a partner; good health; myriad psychological, social, and employment factors; and one's previous sexual activity—what can we say about sexuality and menopause? Surprisingly, there is a lot that you need to know.

Good health contributes to sex vitality because any major debilitating disease can interfere with your feelings of sexuality and your interest in sexual activity. However, it is important to know that individuals with severe disabling diseases can and do remain sexual. Jane Fonda and Jon Voight demonstrate that poignantly in the Academy Award-winning film *Coming Home* in which Voight plays a Vietnam veteran paralyzed from the waist down.

Today, physicians encourage sexual activity even in persons with diseases that previously seemed to mandate avoidance of sexual intercourse. Take heart disease, for example. In previous years, heart patients were advised to give up sex, at least during their early recuperative stages. Today, sexual activity is encouraged as part of their early rehabilitation. Other conditions such as arthritis, back pain, and respiratory diseases can make sexual activity difficult. Yet, physicians are eager to help their patients learn ways to participate in sexual activity that bring pleasure without bringing on painful symptoms or severe shortness of breath.

Sex and the cardiovascular system represent a two-way street; each influences the other. It is known that the act of having sexual intercourse is equivalent to undertaking active exercise. Some researchers have tried to give the range of calories expended during the sex act. Some exercise physiologists have even advised that active sexual intercourse, three times per week, eliminates the need for any other exercise program!

Sex and the Sex Hormones

While sex is doing all these other good things, your sexual response also is increasing the blood flow to your sexual organs. The flow is controlled by a number of factors, but of importance to our discussion of menopause are the contributions of the sex hormones estrogen and progesterone. Estrogen increases the blood flow to the vagina, clitoris, and pelvic muscles. Progestins reduce the blood flow. It is the normal balance between these two powerful hormones that has to be considered.

In 1917, Drs. Stockard and Papanicolaou proved that estrogen increases the thickness of the lining of the vagina. The process is known as *vaginal epithelial buildup.* When you lack estrogen, the vaginal lining thins, as is the case after menopause. It can make penetration during intercourse painful. There is also the interesting matter of enhanced sensation. Research from Yale University shows that as your estrogen level increases, your ability to discriminate sensation on your skin rises. Thus, your ability to feel and respond to touch is better when your estrogen level is high. We know that the more sensitive a woman is to touch, the sexier she feels, and the better the whole process of arousal works.

Masters and Johnson are often quoted for their dictum, "Use it or lose it." Many women want to enjoy sex, but cannot because of pain. Hormone replacement therapy reverses the painful situation by building the vaginal lining and increasing lubrication.

The central and peripheral nervous system is also influenced by the female sex hormones: from the brain down to the sensitive nerve endings in the sex organs and throughout the skin. When women lack estrogen they describe that loss in many ways. It is not unusual for a woman, around the time of menopause, to complain that her clothes do not feel the same on her skin as they formerly did, or that when her sexual partner touches her the sensation is not as enjoyable as it was. The ability to feel or to discriminate between different types of stimuli is enhanced by the presence of estrogen and is diminished when estrogen is lacking. It stands to reason that a woman after the age of menopause, lacking estrogen, is more likely to have a subdued sexual response particularly in the early phases of sexual stimulation.

If a women feels a lack of interest in sex, it may not be caused by a lack of sexual desire (decreased libido), but more likely by a fear of being hurt. The woman who wants to have sex but cannot because she fears pain will be helped remarkably by HRT. It can bring all her tissues back to their normal state. On the other hand, the woman who can have sex comfortably but who doesn't want it may need more help than estrogen alone can provide.

Normal Sexual Behavior After Menopause

What is normal sexual behavior after menopause? Probably anything that satisfies you. There is no "normal" to define. Everyone has completely different needs, goals, determinants of satisfaction, drives, sexual attractions, and sense of attractiveness. Other factors, such as self-esteem, influence sexual vitality as well. These all combine to make us who we are sexually and to determine what we most enjoy and with whom we would seek involvement and participation. You can actually decide for yourself what would determine your normal sexual behavior.

Of course, sexually transmitted diseases, particularly AIDS, are inevitably going to influence your choices concerning what you can undertake sexually. We will discuss this topic in greater detail later in the chapter.

There are a few other specific factors to consider. First, it is becoming more and more unusual for the older woman to be fortunate enough to be in a happy, permanent living arrangement with a partner whom she likes and enjoys. Whether you are heterosexual or homosexual, numerous studies confirm that a satisfactory sex life results when you have an available partner with whom you interact well. For the heterosexual woman, this relationship becomes harder to achieve because of the increased number of women who live longer than men. Both death and divorce result in many women returning to single status. Later in this chapter, we will suggest ways to stay active sexually without cohabitation.

Sexual Problems Around Menopause

For women who experience changes in sexual function during the years immediately preceding and following menopause, the complaints they bring to the physician's office can be divided into five categories:

1. Loss of desire
2. Decreased frequency
3. Painful intercourse

4. Diminished responsiveness
5. Dysfunctions of their male partners

Let's consider these individually, although sometimes these problems may be cumulative for any one couple.

Loss of Desire

Desire is a complex phenomenon. The psychological factors that influence it are extremely important, including the nature of your relationship with your partner. If you experience a loss of desire even though there is still normal hormonal activity in your body, your problem may require deeper evaluation and, perhaps, the help of a sex counselor. At the time of menopause, however, the decline of ovarian hormones often influences the components of sexual desire and arousal. So if your diminished desire is due to a loss of sensory perception through the local and central nervous system, changes in the rate of blood flow, less tension within the muscles, and the decreased ability of the sexual glands to lubricate the vagina, you may be relieved to know that these changes respond very well to HRT. When adequate hormone therapy is introduced, desire and arousal normally return.

Decreased Frequency of Sexual Activity

Again, many factors are at work when you experience decreased frequency of sexual activity, and the majority of them are not hormonal. Most are related to your lifestyle and your relationship with your partner. Together, you need to sort out such issues as fatigue, interest, time, competing activities, or other tensions in the relationship. Do you spend as much "bed time" as television time, or is a too-active social life competing with your sex life? If sex is important equally to you both, you need to work out a mutually satisfactory frequency pattern and set aside the time, create the mood, and satisfy your own and each other's needs whenever possible.

Painful Intercourse

The solution to this problem must include your physician, for this problem is decidedly the easiest to address and, in most instances, it is related to decreased estrogen stimulation of the vaginal canal. Appropriate hormonal replacement almost without exception results in the disappearance of this uncomfortable symptom.

Diminished Responsiveness

This symptom is usually resulting from a decrease in estrogen and the subsequent lack of stimulation of nerves in the pelvic and vaginal area and in the brain itself. Estrogen treatment is of benefit in most instances, and is highly recommended.

Dysfunction of the Male Partner

A surprising finding from research shows that older women have more interest in sex than older men. Possibly one of the biggest problems facing the aging male is his decreased ability to become aroused and, as a result, to obtain or keep an erection for long periods of time. In many cases, this problem can be satisfactorily treated through sexual counseling, which we strongly recommend. Be reassured that even if your male partner is unable to obtain an erection, satisfactory sexual activity can still take place if you are motivated and instructed in other means of sexual gratification.

Achieving sexual satisfaction is largely dependent on your relationship with your partner. You can certainly appreciate the fact that you would not be turned on sexually or able to achieve orgasm if your partner was in pain, disabled, or obviously not enjoying the sexual activity. So it may be that when a man perceives his partner going through menopause; enduring sleep disturbances, hot flashes, and night sweats; feeling unaroused; or suffering painful intercourse, he begins to feel threatened. He may worry that you are losing interest in him because you no longer feel that he is attractive, wanted, or needed. Or he may just be concerned about you and not wish to upset or hurt you by making an issue of your waning sex life. It is true that in a strong relationship one partner suffers from the other partner's ills.

It is important for you both to understand what is happening. Therefore, you should learn about and be willing to explain your problem. If you begin taking hormone therapy and feel relief, let your partner know that you feel better, that your sexuality is intact, and that you are interested in sex again. Knowing these things will often enhance his arousal and change problematic sexual activity back into the healthy and satisfactory sex life that you both enjoy. If you are single, HRT may stimulate you to consider and enjoy a new and invigorating sexual relationship.

Contraception During Perimenopause

Many women say that the best thing about menopause is that they need no longer worry about contraception. It's true! But what is the best method of contraception if you're between thirty-five and menopause? It is interesting to note that what may be a good contraceptive when you are young may not be as good when you are older.

Since women are less fertile in the later reproductive years, a contraceptive method that might have been 90 to 95 percent effective when you were twenty might prove to be almost 100 percent effective when you are 40. A simple barrier method, like the diaphragm, that you were worried about using in your younger years because of its potentially high failure rate, might be a good method later in life. Whatever method you choose, always discuss it with your family practitioner or gynecologist. To give you an overview, however, here are some important facts for women over the age of thirty-five about four different methods of contraception.

The Pill (The Combined Estrogen–Progestin Birth Control Pill)

Beginning in the late 1960s, several major studies were published suggesting that older women who use oral contraceptives (OCs) are at an increased medical risk. Subsequently, women didn't want to take the pill, and physicians would often refrain from prescribing them. Most of these studies concluded that older women using OCs were at higher risk of heart attacks, hypertension, strokes, and overall mortality. But these studies did not look at cigarette smoking, preexisting high blood pressure, and other factors that increase the risk of cardiovascular disease, nor did they differentiate between the various kinds of birth control pills that were being prescribed. Indeed, virtually all the clinical studies were of women using the high-estrogen OCs that have practically disappeared from the market.

The new generation of pills, which have far less hormone in their formulation, are quite different. Another factor, not taken into account, is the potential health benefits of OCs, which include apparently reduced incidences of uterine and ovarian cancer, pelvic inflammatory disease (PID), anemia, and rheumatoid arthritis. Other benefits may include a reduced risk of fibrocystic and other benign breast diseases, improved menstrual cycle control, and relief of PMS, which tends to become more severe after the age of thirty-five. These facts are establishing a strong school of thought, teaching that a woman can continue taking an OC as long as she remains in good health and has no signs of hypertension, late-onset diabetes, uterine lining abnormalities, or other complications. It is also necessary that she have an annual medical screening with a comprehensive physical examination including a blood pressure check, pelvic examination, abdominal palpation, and cholesterol testing. If there is a family history of diabetes, then blood sugar testing is also recommended.

In September 1989, a report from the Harvard Nurses Health Study that appeared in the *Journal of the National Cancer Institute* offered the greatest reassurance. It noted that women over age forty who have used oral contraceptives *do not* have an increased risk of breast cancer, even if they used them for prolonged periods of time.

As women age, however, there are certain other contraindications to taking the pill. A history of cardiovascular disease, liver cancer, breast cancer, diabetes, hypertension, obesity, or uterine fibroids would suggest the need for an alternate method of contraception. Above all, and without exception, smokers should not be taking OCs.

When considering an OC, the pill of choice is one of the new combined, or multiphasic, very low-dose pills. A pill with no more than 35 micrograms of ethinyl estradiol and a consistently low level of progestin, less than one milligram, should be considered. There is actually no persuasive evidence to suggest that one combination pill is better than another as long as you stay with the lowest steroid doses possible that still provide adequate contraceptive protection.

You might consider progestin-only contraceptives, which are being used more often by physicians for their over-forty patients. These are low dose OCs containing no estrogen. As a result, they are appropriate for midlife women with gall bladder disease or impaired liver function who would not be candidates for a combined OC. These particular pills are very rarely prescribed for younger women because of their higher failure rate (up to 2 percent) in preventing pregnancy and also because they tend to cause irregular bleeding due to their lack of estrogen. It would appear that the failure rate declines to about 1 percent in women over thirty-five and that older women are also less likely to experience irregular bleeding as a side effect. If all of the above precautions, indications, and clinical observations are carefully followed, older women can safely take birth control pills until the age of menopause and then simply switch to one of the alternate estrogen replacement therapies allowing for a continuum of birth control pill contraception until postmenopausal HRT begins. Of course, the kind of estrogen differs after menopause (see chapter 5).

Intrauterine Devices

The intrauterine device (IUD) is an exceptionally good method of contraception despite the adverse publicity it receives. The design, particularly the monofilamentous tail, of the modern types of IUD that are available (like the Copper T or the Progestasert), and the fact that IUDs are being recommended for women over thirty-five who have completed their families, makes this population the most ideal for using this method of contraception. An IUD can be inserted after age thirty-five and changed every four to five years, making it an unobtrusive, effective, and inexpensive birth control method. The risks associated with the IUD include uterine perforation, which is rare, and pelvic inflammatory disease, which is also rare, particularly in stable monogamous relationships. The failure rates with IUDs in women who are over thirty-five are extremely low and the removal of the device is usually very easy. The IUD is a method that should be considered.

Barrier and Chemical Methods

Methods such as the diaphragm, condom, and spermicides offer realistic alternatives for many couples, given the older age of the individual and her consequent decline in fertility. These methods are not failproof, and it is wise to consider potential risks of pregnancy. The condom and spermicide (if it contains nonoxynol-9 as its active ingredient) are increasingly popular because they may prevent transmission of the AIDS virus. The greater availability and the wide acceptance of the condom makes it a perfectly satisfactory contraceptive choice for women over thirty-five.

Sterilization

Sterilization remains the most frequently chosen method of contraception for women age thirty-five and older. Failure rates are low, but remember this method is permanent and should be undertaken only after you make a well-thought-out decision that you will not later regret. Newer methods of female sterilization have focused on achieving safe, simple tubal occlusion created by placing a silastic (an inert plastic) ring, or clip, on the fallopian tube through an instrument called a laparoscope. It is a short surgical procedure that has few complications and is widely accepted by women.

But What about AIDS?

We are in a new age with a new problem. The advent of AIDS has changed sexual mores drastically. The fact that medical science does not have the answers to this devastating illness is distressing and makes our ability to advise anyone on how to avoid AIDS extremely difficult. If you are in a monogamous relationship with no outside sexual contact by either partner, you have no cause for fear. But if you are not sure of that, or if you wish to enter into a new relationship, we understand the real possibility of danger that gives rise to your fears.

Evaluation of epidemiologic information about AIDS suggests that women currently in the perimenopausal or postmenopausal years show an extremely low incidence of AIDS. This finding may apply to the group as a whole, but how do you interpret it as an individual? With great caution!

Because men and women are both fearful of AIDS, they are willing to talk about it. Communication between you and your partner-to-be is of paramount importance. You need to discuss your sexuality and sexual history and raise the question of a meaningful, honest, one-to-one relationship that you hope will last, at least for a while. Allow your relationship to develop, and when sexual activity becomes a possibility, do not hesitate to discuss your fear of AIDS.

The simplest way to be sure that your partner is not going to infect you is for both of you to have an AIDS screening test. It does put an end to spontaneous first-time sex. But, if it is going to reassure you as you develop a longstanding monogamous relationship, then have the test done. The chances of receiving a positive result are very low; the chances of reassuring you are extremely high.

Without AIDS testing, and the knowledge that your partner is going to remain faithful to you alone, there are other steps that should be used in all future sexual encounters. Safer sex will not only help prevent exposure to AIDS but will help safeguard you against the whole range of so-called sexually transmitted diseases (STDs). Safer sex allows all your usual activities and feelings, as long as there is no exchange of body fluids. It essentially means using condoms during vaginal and oral sex with any partner that has not been proven to be free and clear of AIDS, and avoiding direct contact with any body fluids.

This new sexual environment places a new and heavy responsibility on you. Only you can ask the right questions of your potential sexual partner. And you must ask! Your health and your life may depend on it. Otherwise, your only alternative at this time is to choose celibacy, which may not be your preference. We suggest that you ask the right questions, insist on honest and open answers, and only then permit the relationship to move forward sexually.

What about Masturbation?

In the absence of an acceptable partner, masturbation is a reasonable and appropriate source of sexual enjoyment as well as a method of releasing sexual tension. At midlife and thereafter, women may choose this form of sexual release as the shortage of available men gives way to the general shortage of men in an aging population. Masturbation may also be the sexual outlet of choice, over and above available partners. Masturbation is also a good way of getting started for women who, because of estrogen depletion, experience arousal too slowly to begin sexual activity at the same time as a mate. It is also a loving way to express sexuality for men or women during the illness of either partner or in instances when the desired amount of sexual activity differs for each partner.

There is no right and no wrong when it comes to sex. Society's very recent acceptance of individual sexual preferences has also lifted the taboo on masturbation. Just as children need to be assured that there is nothing wrong with masturbation, so older persons need to know that it is not an improper activity for them. Although there is less disapproval of masturbation today than in prior times, there is still significant discomfort with the issue. However, if we agree that sexuality is basic to life, then masturbation must be included as one of our natural sexual outlets. According to one study, nearly half of the women questioned indicated that they masturbated in their fifties, and this amount decreased to about one-third of the women at age seventy and over. Two-thirds of the men involved in this study masturbated in their fifties and this amount dropped to 47 percent at age seventy or greater. Those achieving orgasm ranged from 83 percent of the women at age fifty to 74 percent when they reached their seventies and beyond. In their fifties, 91 percent of the men reached orgasm. At age seventy and later, 73 percent of the men who masturbated reached orgasm.

Mutual masturbation is another way to enhance your sex life when you want to, or when other possibilities are limited because of illness or injury. It involves each partner giving each other pleasure until such time as they are both ready to join in whatever way is possible for them.

The techniques for masturbation are as varied and individual as what brings you satisfaction and pleasure. Do not be afraid to experiment. Self-experience and self-pleasure are valuable safe sex techniques. You do not actually need to have sexual relations with another person to feel sexually fulfilled.

In the study by Masters and Johnson that we mentioned earlier, it was found that each of the female volunteers masturbated differently. So you need to try and see what feels good to you. You may use your fingers and hands in caressing motions in whatever position feels best. Some women stroke or press, covering their entire genital area, whereas others find that stimulating the clitoris feels best. Hands and fingers can provide intense stimulation by stroking and rubbing the external genitals, by the fingers' gentle thrusting motion in the vagina, or by a combination of both. There is no preferred way of self-stimulation; only personal preferences apply.

Vibrators also provide stimulation and excitement to many sensitive areas of the body and can be used in many ways. They come in both electric and battery-operated models and in shapes as different as women are unique. They also sidestep the old taboo of not touching oneself for women who find it is a lingering problem. These are available for purchase in pharmacies and most department stores, as well as offered in catalogues too numerous to mention.

Jacuzzi jets or hand-held shower heads playing directly on the clitoris can offer sexual pleasure, and for some women so does the crossbar of a bicycle or the back of a horse when riding. Do not be afraid to try to seek sexual pleasure by yourself or to engage in a satisfying fantasy life that may stimulate you in different ways by "dream" imaging. Erotic books, movies, and videotapes may also be used to heighten your sexual excitement. Just remember, there would not be so many erotic items available if they were not in use. If you are not sure of how to start your process of experimentation, there are many good books available that offer specific instructions and techniques for masturbation, such as L.G. Barbach's, *For Yourself: The Fulfillment of Female Sexuality* (New York, Anchor/Doubleday, 1976) and *Sex Is Not Simple* by Stephen B. Levine (Ohio, Ohio Publishing Co., 1988). You can also try to find a support group for women that deals with sexuality.

Enhancing Sexuality

As with other compelling factors in your life, your sexuality is up to you. Whether you are considering partner or solo sex, there are a number of ways in which you may want to modify your behavior to enhance your sexuality safely. These may include, but are not limited to, the following:

1. If you are losing sensation and sexuality because of menopause, see your physician, have a physical evaluation, and see if you can consider HRT.
2. Take a personal physical evaluation naked in front of a full-length mirror.
   Are you comfortable with what you see? _____
   If not, are you willing to diet and exercise to recreate a healthier, sexier you? _____
3. Look at yourself as you get ready to get into bed with or without a partner. Do you look good to you? _____
   If not, what is wrong? _____
   Freshly bathed or showered? _____
   Pretty/sexy nightclothes? _____
   Combed hair? _____
   Scrubbed face? _____
   Good attitude? _____
   (Notice we did not determine what is sexy or attractive. Here again, take note of your personal preferences.)
4. Is the setting you've created conducive to your need for a sexual activity? _____
5. What about the ambience: soft music or erotic videotape, soft light, candlelight, no light? It's up to you, but is it right for you?

6. Has the time preceding this been pleasant and conducive to sexual activity or has it been rife with unpleasantness and controversy?

7. If a partner is involved, are you both on the same wavelength: Have you discussed what you want so you won't be disappointed? _____

8. Is there more that you can do to let your partner know you are ready to engage in sexual activity? _____
9. Have you done all you can to try to ensure that you will not be disturbed by the telephone, doorbell, kids? _____
10. Can you rid yourself of all of the self-limiting concerns that preclude your total involvement in sex? _____
11. If the sexual encounter is unsatisfactory for whatever reason, are you prepared to accept it, learn from it, and set the stage for a successful next encounter? _____
12. Do you feel loved? _____

Your responses to these suggestions and questions will determine for you what you need to do to get the most and the best out of your sexual activity. They should serve as a guide for finding out what you want and how to get it.

Just as there is no definition of "normal" for sexuality and no recipe for enjoyable sexual activity, there is no prescription for good mood- and mind-setting behavior. When it comes to successful sex, your own uniqueness will determine what is right and pleasurable for you. Just remember that enjoying your sexuality is something you can continue to do for as long as you live.

A Word About Late Pregnancy

It may strike you as odd that we include pregnancy in a chapter on sexuality and aging. We assure you that it belongs here. We often need to respond to, "How does my age impact on my chances for a healthy and successful pregnancy?" It is a question asked of obstetricians as more and more women are choosing to conceive after the age of thirty-five. It is not always easy to do because fertility rates decrease with age, but it happens with increasing frequency as fertility treatment becomes more sophisticated and successful.

You may be interested to know that prior to 1975, the peak years for women to have babies were between their twentieth and twenty-ninth birthdays. Then, at the height of the "baby boom," in 1975, the birth rate in the United States started downward. The major reason for the decline was the change in contraceptive practices. Many more married women of childbearing age were using contraception in the 1980s than in the 1960s. (Married women between ages thirty-five and forty-four use contraception less often than younger wives. When they do, they tend either to end fertility permanently, through sterilization, or to rely on nonmedical methods.)

Recently, however, the downward trend ended, as the large group of "baby boomers" began having babies at age thirty-five or older. "Late pregnancies" increased by a whopping 37 percent. This switch is the subject of several studies of women over age thirty-five, designed to learn whether there is an increased risk associated with pregnancy, childbirth, or the period of confinement after labor for this growing group of women.

Recently reported results suggest that the risk of some problems in pregnancy may increase in midlife and that hypertension, diabetes, preeclampsia (toxemia of late pregnancy that includes hypertension, albuminuria, and edema), and premature labor may be more common in women who give birth after the age of forty. Much of the time, however, these complications can be taken care of medically and usually do not increase mortality.

The increase in diabetes is understandable. We know that there is an increase in diabetes mellitus with age, and so this problem is more likely to appear in women over thirty-five. Yet, even with this increase in incidence of diabetes and hypertension, modern prenatal care should assure normal results for mother and baby as long as mother is healthy when the pregnancy begins. However, women with medical complications, such as chronic hypertension or diabetes mellitus *before* pregnancy, may find that these conditions tend to be aggravated. They could affect baby's health and survival.

A frequently asked question is whether women over thirty-five are more likely to have smaller babies. The answer is "no." According to various studies, there is an increased birth weight in babies delivered by older women.

Delivery itself is another matter. Generally, there are fewer vaginal deliveries after the age of forty. This increase in cesarean sections is apparent in most of the medical literature.

After the baby is born, there might be an increased risk to the mother of fever due to infection, or of blood clots and possibly pulmonary emboli. The incidence of these complications is not dramatic, however, and doctors generally can recognize and treat these problems effectively. As far as the baby is concerned, chromosomal abnormality is one of the major worries of women having later pregnancies. A direct correlation between the age of the mother and chromosomal abnormality does exist, particularly in the number of Down syndrome infants that are liveborn. At age twenty-five there is one Down syndrome birth in 1,200; this statistic increases to one in 365 at age thirty-five; it jumps to one in 32 at age forty-five.

When all other chromosomal abnormalities are included, the risks are even higher. A review of middle-trimester amniocentesis data reveals that the risk increases from 1.3 percent at age thirty-five to 1.9 percent at age forty, and to almost 10 percent beyond age forty.

The most recent best-controlled hospital-based studies suggest that women of advanced maternal age delivering under optimum conditions may be at no higher risk for adverse outcome than pregnancies in younger patients. There once was a term, the *elderly prima gravida,* which referred to a woman who had never had a child before age thirty-five. The term is obsolete! We believe that in the absence of underlying medical disorders, and assuming modern obstetric care including prenatal diagnosis, advanced age in itself only minimally increases pregnancy risks.

·10·

Men and Menopause

Why do some middle-aged men stray from their wives toward younger women? Why do they buy expensive sports cars? Why do a few of them just seem to go to pieces at midlife? These questions inevitably lead to the eternal one: Is there a male menopause? Do men go through hormonal changes that create physical, emotional, and behavioral changes?

Hormonal Aspects of Male Menopause

Over the years, researchers have tried to determine whether there is a male equivalent of the female menopause. As you know, the female menopause is the result of the ovary running out of eggs and being unable to produce the female hormones estrogen and progesterone. Investigators have evaluated the male testis to see whether it goes through the same kind of changes and whether it, like the ovary, reduces production of its sex hormone, testosterone.

The testis is to man what the ovary is to woman—a gland with two express functions: reproduction and hormone production. The most remarkable difference between them is that the man's testis somehow maintains its ability to produce spermatozoa throughout life, whereas the woman's ovary never produces a single new egg from the time she is born. So the healthy male is able to father children as long as he lives, and the female's reproductive life ends at menopause. Was this apparent inequity nature's way of protecting the species, assuring that a woman would live long enough to nurture her young inasmuch as she could only conceive while she had enough years left to care for them? Or is it simply an unfair quirk of nature whose purpose, if any, we do not yet understand?

There has been remarkably little good scientific evaluation of the change in male hormone production throughout the male life cycle. The best studies were conducted only in the last decade. The results suggest that the male hormone, testosterone, exhibits a characteristic pattern throughout a man's life. Its levels first peak during the male's intrauterine life, at about fourteen to sixteen weeks into the pregnancy; then the level begins to drop. There is another brief peak after a boy baby is born; then the testosterone level drops and remains low until puberty. At that time there is a sharp increase in the blood level of testosterone that continues from puberty until a man is in his mid-fifties, or later. From then on, there is a slow decrease in testosterone levels.

Another important aspect to consider is that both men and women have some hormone of the opposite sex circulating in their blood. So when the blood testosterone levels decrease in men, there is a relative increase in their estrogen levels as they age.

Investigators have found that in the older man, there is a decrease in the actual number of cells that produce sex hormones. However, there is very little data analyzing the sperm of men as they age. Generally, it seems that sperm counts remain unaltered. If we take into account that sexual activity slows down, then sperm production may actually be decelerating with age. Parallel with the decreased sperm production is a reduction in the sperm's ability to move forward actively (motility) and to get to its destination.

Despite these changes, a man tends to remain hormonally and reproductively normal until he enters his late fifties, or even his early sixties. At that time, some changes occur in testicular function, but the process of change for the male is very slow, and there is no comparison with the abrupt changes that occur in women.

Another fact to consider in exploring the idea of whether or not men undergo a male menopause is that male life expectancy is shorter than that of the female, and the slight reduction in testicular function tends to occur in the last years of his life. Thus, a man is potentially virile and potent—if his health and all other aspects remain equal—until close to the end of life. So these changes are more subtle than a woman's and often do not make serious inroads on a man's life.

What Are Possible Symptoms of Male Menopause?
What does occur when men are around middle-age? Findings have suggested that some older men complain of reduced libido or sexual potency, increased fatigue, decreasing productivity and concentration, sweating, tachycardia (excessively rapid heartbeat), skin atrophy, sleep disturbances, anxiety, and depression. There also have been reports of male hot flashes! The clustering of these symptoms around the ages of forty-five through sixty ushered the phrase *male climacteric syndrome* into vogue almost fifty years ago.

The truth is that there is no such thing as the male climacteric syndrome when evaluated in hormonal or psychopathological terms. There are minor chemical changes that do occur but are relatively insignificant. In one study, 10,000 male outpatients claiming to be suffering from the male climacteric were evaluated statistically. No age-related increase in the frequency of depression, fatigueability, and decreased activity was found. The generally accepted conclusion is that certain symptoms do increase in men of advancing age, and these affect sex, memory, and sleep. However, they do not cluster between the ages of forty-five to sixty, but instead just continue to increase slowly with advancing age, and there is no justification for calling any syndrome the male climacteric. These changes are age-related, not sex-related. Since there are no menses, and therefore no cessation of menses in men, the term *male menopause* is not valid.

So What Is It That They Call the Male Menopause?

Although there is technically no male menopause on which to blame the rather peculiar behavior some men exhibit as they pass the age of fifty, many female patients say that they are confused by odd behavior in their middle-aged spouse, male family members, friends, or co-workers. If we accept that there are no specific hormonal changes and no real male menopause, how do we explain this unusual behavior?

First, let us consider some of the unusual behaviors. It is more than a cliché that some men in mid-life crisis give up their conservative Oldsmobile for an expensive Ferrari, or move out of their home, leaving their wife and family for a woman half their age. You see these men all over the place, looking out of place as they relate romantically to women the ages of their daughters or nieces. The occurrence repeats itself too often to be ignored. Why is it happening?

Does it result from a man's need for outside recognition of his accomplishments, power, and attractiveness? Is it a salve to soothe a sense of failure or dissatisfaction with his life? Is he trying to escape from facing his own mortality? Does the recognition and fear of aging and thoughts of diminished skills and physical prowess lead some men into a phase of frantic and erratic behavior?

Probably all the above! On the one hand, a highly successful man may feel that he has peaked and worries about his future growth and development. Where can he go now? He knows that since he has reached the peak, he has to fight to stay there. He has reached a serious period of transition in his life and is unsure of his future direction. These situations differ for each man and seem to be more of a problem for some than for others. Yet our social scientists tell us that for each man a time of personal evaluation arrives. For many, it is a manageable thought-provoking time. For others, it is incredibly frightening. The man of awareness and reason will value the reappraisal that is appropriate to this period of life. Others, unable to deal with this time of personal questioning and uncertainty, turn emotional turmoil into a series of dramatic life changes that temporarily mask their discomfort.

This time of life may be experienced differently by men and women because of how they perceive themselves and their needs at midlife. It may be that men have a crisis of performance, whereas women suffer a crisis of appearance. Some men seek reassurance by continually surrounding themselves with material objects to serve as reminders of success. Sometimes a man seeks a new relationship with a younger woman. A young adoring mistress may boost his ego. But, what of loyalty at home?

Is a man's home life not living up to his needs as he perceives them? Can he move easily from his sophisticated dynamic work environment to his more static home life comfortably? Can he continue to enjoy, even relish, the comfortable relationship with his lifelong mate or is he seeking titillating renewal with a younger, or a different, woman? Can he age comfortably with his home life intact? Many men can; some men just cannot; other men seem to want to have both: their Mrs. and their mistresses.

The fear of aging and death seems to be much worse for men than for women, perhaps with some justification. Statistics prove that men die at a younger age than women. They experience more heart attacks, and they may actually be the weaker sex! We know that around the age of fifty, women are experiencing many great changes in family and friend relationships. They also are often changing or leaving jobs, and if the children no longer live at home and the "empty nest" is a reality, they may have more time for hobbies, sports, or just for themselves. For some women this change is welcome; for others it is fraught with the stress of readjustment.

A man has an even bigger problem to face. He has to watch as his male peers, friends, old school mates, business partners, competitors, and family members are struck down around him with diagnoses of diabetes, heart disease, cancer, and other medical problems. These events bombard him again and again with the fact that life—his life—is finite. The vulnerable male, so bombarded with news of illness and death, reads the obituaries and attends the funerals in ever-increasing numbers and his thoughts fill with the question, "Is that all there is?"

Although women experience illness and death among their family members, friends, and coworkers, too, somehow they seem to handle these matters with greater equanimity. In men, these experiences seem to result in conflict as they think about and fear the changes occurring within their own life. They confront their own circumstances, their own life patterns, and their own mortality. Part of this "change of life" for them is also influenced by the changes happening to their partners. Maybe these changes are worse for some men because of how they were nurtured. Whereas women can freely express emotion, men were often told not to cry. So, they don't cry at the loss of father, mother, or even their youth. When men's emotions become bottled tightly inside themselves, the bottled-up mess may eventually explode.

Sometimes the fallout can be highly productive. It can drive them toward a new career, to a new and exciting activity, or to new levels of intimacy with a much-loved partner. Or it can lead to disaster—to a broken marriage, a failed business, a sense of worthlessness, feelings of inadequacy, and even suicide. Sometimes it manifests itself as a need for more "toys," more trips, more women, more of anything that says to them, "You are still virile, you are still exciting, you still turn me on, you are still young!"

Young is the important word: It is the important feeling. It means growth, potential, and promise. It offers the hope of immortality!

Are Men's Problems Complicated
by Women's Menopause?

We live inside our own mind and body and look out from the inside. It may be that the only time a man looks at his own outside or studies his mirror image is early in the morning when he shaves. Yet, what of his partner who sees him as he is? What of their relationship, which may be significantly altered by his aging? Perhaps the man returns home in the evening and to his wife he looks tired and slightly puffy; he needs a shave, and although the gray in his hair lends distinction, she sees him and knows him as the age that he is, which is fine, because she is aware of her aging appearance as well. He, in contrast, may perceive his wife's appearance only in relation to *her* age and how *she* looks. He may never relate it to his *own* aging self. When he does, it shocks the daylights out of him!

Some people seem to think that appearance is the main attraction for men, whereas women seek sensitivity and intellectual depth. Often, in some mature relationships, the wife sees her husband as powerful and bright. When the husband sees his aging wife, however, he may see in her changed appearance a reflection of his own altered image and see the enemy—old age—approaching. This perception is not the wife's fault; it is merely a fact of life. Sometimes a man leaves his wife, and the only explanation he can give her is, "When I'm with you I feel old." It's a tragic response to years of loyalty and commitment, yet the need to run surges forth from deep within the man. It is comprised of unexpressed fears and emotions that have been buried so deep within him for so long that even he cannot tap their source. In an odd way, and without knowing why, his answer may be close to the whole truth.

What else about his partner reminds him of change that is scary? Apart from her somewhat changed external appearance, there are behavioral changes that occur in direct relation to her body's biochemical changes that may also influence his perception. The thinning of her vaginal lining and painful intercourse may begin to intrude upon their sexual relationship. Changing bed linen or clothing in the middle of the night becomes the result of sweaty hot flashes instead of steamy sex. Add the fact that the man may be having an increasing problem with obtaining and maintaining an erection. Imagine the hesitation he feels at even trying to have intercourse with his wife when he realizes that she is enduring discomfort. They both know that sex should be enjoyable, not physically or emotionally painful. So he may just stop trying to relate sexually to her, and she may not object.

Meanwhile during the male's daily activities at work or at play, if he is exuding the charisma of money or power, he may attract younger women. They make him feel good by subconsciously enabling him to project a longer and healthier future for himself. With problems at home that he doesn't understand or relate to, he enters into a relationship that he did not initially chase or choose.

It is fair, then, to say that one part of the male's awareness of the problems in his life is triggered by a woman's menopause. This is not to lay responsibility on a woman for a man's crisis, but it is to say that a woman's changes in midlife are noticed by a man, and he cannot help but begin to examine the changes that are occurring in his own life at this time.

Sadly, much of the marital disillusionment, discord, and dissolution that occur when otherwise good marriages become shaky, around the time of menopause, are fully preventable. The problems must be recognized for what they are. You can work through the problems once you understand them, rather than abandoning the relationship or continuing the infidelity. The solution to the problems lies in open, honest communication.

How Can the Perimenopausal Woman Help Keep Her Relationship Strong?

There is plenty that the perimenopausal woman can do to secure her relationship with her mate, if that is what she desires. All the effort revolves around one word: *recognition.* First, recognize that this time in life may hold potential problems for you and your partner. Next, recognize what is going on in both your lives; understand the dynamics of what you are doing and what you are feeling and try to understand his as well. Only then can you recognize and appreciate the choices you have for minimizing the possible negative effects of midlife on both of you. Obviously, you cannot prevent the aging process. The process of living makes the process of aging inevitable. Let's concentrate on the process of living!

We can delay many of the consequences of aging. The Utian Menopause Management Program shows you how to recognize and optimize factors of the aging process. It incorporates an action plan to make the most of midlife and the years that follow.

What Must a Man Do for Himself?

Recognition is the operative word here, too! A problem must be recognized before a solution can be created. You've often heard it said, "If it ain't broken, don't fix it." Well, a corollary might be, "How can you even begin to fix it if you don't recognize that it is damaged?"

It is important for men to know that there are active steps that they can take to find greater satisfaction in their middle years, enhance the joy of life, and prevent relationships from damage.

We suggest the following four-point plan:

1. Get your partner to read chapter 2, this chapter, and the last chapter of the book. It would be even better if he read the whole book, but settle for these few pages. This brief read should help him to recognize problems that men can suffer in midlife and see that prevention is possible.

2. Encourage your mate to express emotion. The male at midlife, or better yet before, should do an emotional inventory. He needs to sit back in a comfortable chair, gaze at the ceiling, and try to work out how he feels about his life and his accomplishments. He needs to develop a life-satisfaction checklist. His stated purpose must be an honest evaluation of his set of values. What is important to him? Does he need/want to give up the hectic social chase for intellectual and academic pursuits? He should ask himself whether he is angry with you for reasons that have nothing to do with the aging process. What is getting in the way of your growing old happily together?

3. Accept the fact that hormonal changes in your man are not occurring with any drama and that they are not to blame for his emotional changes. In other words, if he is otherwise healthy, male midlife crisis cannot be the fault of physical/hormonal phenomena. Help him search for other reasons.

4. Recruit your mate as your partner in following the Utian Menopause Management Program. It is just as important for him to undertake a healthy diet, begin an appropriate exercise program, and look

at himself in the mirror more than once each day. He, too, needs a reassuring medical examination, professional dental care, a good haircut and styling, and well-fitted clothing.

We would feel the joy of true contribution if this book could serve as a catalyst for a couple sitting down and discussing where they are in their lives as individuals and as a couple, and how they feel about it. Two loving people who recognize that aging is a natural phenomenon will discover that there are things that each can do to excite and enhance the other's life and the life that they share. It would be wonderful if each person, instead of being reactive to the other, could become restorative. It's as simple and as complex as saying, "I know how you feel, I care about how you feel, and I will try to help you to feel better."

·11·

Teeth to Toes: Total Body Care

We have explored the ways you can take care of your "inside" self: medically, therapeutically, nutritionally, physically, sexually, and psychologically. In this chapter we will discuss the *outside* of you: what others see when they look at you. As all the inside work you do has outside effects, so the outside work improves the inside. You feel better when you look good.

When You're Smiling . . .

Laugh and the world laughs with you, smile and it sees your teeth. Good teeth are important throughout life and a real benefit at midlife. You can manage to keep your own teeth for life with proper daily cleaning and flossing and professional care at least twice a year. You can avoid the dental problems that start around midlife such as receding gums, change in color as the tooth enamel thins, and half a lifetime of staining. From puberty to menopause, estrogen helped to maintain your healthy gums and jawbones. Without estrogen, the same tissue and bone changes that we described in chapter 5 begin to occur. Gingivectomy, a procedure to repair gum after periodontal disease, has typically been called a woman's midlife oral surgery procedure. It becomes necessary when the gums are weakened by disease or the jawbones shrink and, as a result, teeth become loose.

Daily cleaning, flossing before bed, regular checkups with professional cleaning to remove plaque, and replacement of missing teeth can help you avoid this midlife trap. Although you can expect to keep your teeth longer because of fluoridation in the water (if it is available

163

in your area), you still have to combat the sticky surface plaque that causes disease. Flossing once in a while doesn't help. Plaque is back at its destructive job within twenty-four hours.

Did you know that a whole new branch of dentistry called cosmetic dentistry can also dramatically improve your smile? The last decade has brought forth more and more ways to make you look better. Dentists can close spaces or gaps between teeth; change the size and shape of teeth; repair chipped, broken, and discolored teeth; and bleach teeth.

Dentists can also change unsightly old silver fillings to "tooth-colored" ones. Today, besides caps, there are other ways to improve the looks of teeth. Just a few years ago, cosmetic bonding became technologically available. It is a process by which a new surface can be laminated over your own tooth to give it a newer, whiter coat. With the new resin-bonding materials, your teeth can suddenly become younger looking. The latest development in dentistry is porcelain laminate. Used to cover your front teeth after they are etched, or roughed up a bit for better contact but not pared down as for caps, porcelain laminates slip-cover the fronts of your front teeth, covering any unsightliness.

Hair Harmony

There is no need for your hair to look less than wonderfully luxuriant at midlife. It's true that individual hair shafts begin to thin and fade and become dryer when you are about forty. Changes in your hair after menopause generally are the result of hormonal changes. You can counter these changes by giving your crowning glory better care, and a new and more flattering cut and style. You can try to stop drying it further with electrical tools, harsh chemicals, poor diet, poor circulation, and too much exposure to the elements.

If you love your hair, it won't disappoint you. True female baldness is a rare problem; it usually has a genetic base, if it occurs. Hair loss, when caused by disease, will usually regrow and be as healthy as it was before. Since you were very young, you have been losing 50 to 120 hairs each day. Thus, about 30,000 hairs per year are replaced by new ones. As we age, sometimes the replacement process is slower. Usually, past forty, the replacement hairs are a lighter, or faded, version of the ones you lost. The texture and consistency may also change. If you crash diet regularly, your hair will rebel against the lack of nutrition by becoming dry and brittle. If you combine your internal abuse with normal aging changes, and then add external abuses of overstyling or improper coloring or perming techniques, you can't expect your hair to care for you.

First, you should know that everyone eventually turns gray. We lose pigment as we age, and by fifty, half of the population is gray-haired. Well-cared-for gray hair can look chic, stunning, and appealing depending on its condition and styling. Frizzy, dry, flyaway gray is not flattering. A long bob of gray hair is just too much of a good thing. A shorter blunt cut, good conditioning to make it shine, and a color rinse to heighten, deepen, or lighten the gray, if necessary, is all you need.

On the other hand, if gray is not your favorite color, change it early. When you find you are spending more time jerking gray hairs from your head than washing it, it's time to consider color. If you like the gray coming in naturally and appreciate the salt and pepper stage, leave it alone. If you are thinking about coloring your hair eventually, skip the salt and pepper stage. Simply go from your hair color back to your hair color, by gradually adding color as your natural color fades. You can enjoy your hair color for a lifetime. Did you always want to find out whether blondes have more fun, or redheads are more exciting? Then switch colors, but first make sure the color you choose is flattering to you. Often a change in hair color means a change in makeup palette. We will cover cosmetics later in this chapter.

For hair-care harmony, use as few electrical appliances on your hair as possible. If you use a dryer, keep it at least six inches away from your head. Turn off the dryer just before your hair is completely dry. If you use rollers, curlers, or bobby pins, don't pull on the hair excessively. Use quality hair-care products that are right for your type of hair. Practice good nutrition and meet the recommended daily requirements for vitamins A, B, C, D, and E, which may have especially good effects on your hair. HRT helps as well. Cover your hair in the sun and wind and rinse it after you swim to get rid of pool chemicals.

Removing Body Hair

As you get into midlife, the hormonal changes in your body express themselves in many ways. As estrogen diminishes, male hormones increase and you may be faced with excess hair on your face, chest, or abdomen. It's all a part of the normal aging process, but you don't need to keep it.

There are several hair removal methods that work well. Although shaving does not make hair grow back thicker, it only lasts a day or two. Plucking, or tweezing, is a good way to get rid of a hair here and there on the face. Make sure your tweezers are clean by wiping them with alcohol. If you prefer, you can try bleaching the offending hairs, which will make them less conspicuous. There are many depilatory creams on the market, but check for sensitivity or allergic response by trying a product in a small unobtrusive place, such as the inside of your forearm. To get slower regrowth, you can try waxing. There are hot and cold waxes on the market and many salons offer this service. The longest delay of regrowth is achieved with electrolysis, which must be done by a trained technician. An electrically driven needle kills the hair down to the root before plucking it out. This procedure is expensive and somewhat uncomfortable, and it may take many sessions to remove all the hair from a small area. The cost of electrolysis varies greatly from state to state. If you are considering electrolysis, make sure you locate a reputable licensed practitioner. A referral from a dermatologist is usually a good way to find one.

Saving Your Skin

We have covered the effects of estrogen on the skin, the largest organ of the body. You can review them in chapters 3 and 5. Estrogen thickens the skin. Additionally, it is the effect of estrogen on the exocrine glands that helps to keep the skin moisturized, plumped up, and smooth. Lacking estrogen, dryness results.

The skin also shows the results of aging in many ways that can be flattering, softening harsh features, and showing inner character. The deeper layer of the skin loses its moisture and elasticity, and so it shrinks. The outer skin, or epidermis, is now looser than the inner layer and so it hangs, or creases. How and when this aging happens depends on many factors. Your genetic makeup plays its part as does whether you had acne or another skin condition, and whether you smoke. The skin also has slower circulation so it may become blotchy, with broken capillaries, perhaps the result of hormonal ups and downs. The skin becomes lighter and rougher-textured from enlarged pores. Exercise provides help because it nourishes the skin and creates moisture.

Why do many women get upset every time a new wrinkle appears? Perhaps self-esteem gets in the way of reality. In your thirties, you laugh off the first laugh lines or crow's-feet that spring up around the outer edges of the eyes, or the frown lines that mark the forehead. When you are fifty or more, the accumulation of sun, normal loss of elasticity, and the pull of gravity may cause the little vertical "stitches" that run around the upper lip. The skin may droop slightly under the chin, the jaw line may gather two small pouches on either side, and the skin on the neck may slacken.

You have more than twenty years between laugh lines and lip stitches. If you limit your exposure to the sun, protect against the sun when exposed, and apply moisturizer daily (many are prepared with sunscreen added for protection), you can delay the aging of the skin by many years. Once it begins, there is no cosmetic product that can rid you of wrinkles, age spots, or facial blemishes, although some can give you a mini-lift for a couple of hours.

Retin-A, the new "dream cream" on the market, is showing good results in removing tiny surface wrinkles and lightening brown spots. It is a product that may retard the effects of photoaging of your skin (the aging caused by sun exposure, which shows up as wrinkled, yellowish, rough, lax, and leathery skin with age spots and sometimes with fine veins that mar cheeks and nose). Before considering Retin-A, a visit to your dermatologist is essential for examination, explanation, prescription, and follow-up care.

Aging skin does not bother all women, and it need not bother you. If you can value the outward charm of aging along with the wisdom of your experience, then you will see the beauty and dignity of aging as you are. We are reminded of famous artist Georgia O'Keeffe, who died in her nineties and whose face grew more beautiful with age. We imagine she used a good moisturizer and little else on that interesting face.

If you want to change your skin in a more lasting way, we will be describing plastic surgery possibilities later in this chapter.

Nail Care

Nails and hair depend on good nutrition, exercise, and hormone balance for their health. They are made of keratin, and although there is nothing you can apply to make them grow faster, they will grow forever if they are not severely damaged. Nails also tell medical tales. Conditions like anemia, thyroid disorders, and protein deficiency from crash dieting show up in their thinning, cracking, and color distortion. See your dermatologist if problems with your nails persist.

Healthy-looking nails are neatly trimmed and filed. The cuticle is there to protect your nail, so pushing it back gently seems to be a better idea than cutting it. You should remove all hangnails using clean manicure scissors or nippers. It is also a good idea to protect your nails by wearing the appropriate work gloves.

You may prefer short nails to long ones, light polish to dark or bright polish, square tips to oval ones. If your hands are very wrinkled or age spotted, you may find that medium short nails, with paler or clear polish, may make your hands look younger.

Toenails should be cut straight across. A typical problem nail is one that has become too thick, which may occur when the toe nails are too long, or from tight shoes, flat feet, or fungus infection. Well-groomed feet not only look good but they make you step lighter and feel better. If you can, midlife is the time to treat yourself to pedicures, either at home or at the beauty salon. And they are so relaxing!

Commonsense Cosmetics

Earlier we said that the skin becomes lighter and its texture changes somewhat as you age. Thus, makeup that has always looked good on you may look odd. Either it is too dark or too light or too bold. You should experiment with color. A good way to begin is to schedule an appointment with a professional makeup artist. (Makeup artists are usually available at the cosmetic counters of department stores.) Without explaining in detail what is bothering you, see what makeup products and colors they choose for you.

For makeup to work for you, it all has to work together. Midlife is usually not the time for makeup extremes, even if you could get away with them in your younger years. The natural look is beautiful and makeup should serve as enhancement, not camouflage. Consumers spend billions of dollars a year on cosmetics. If you support this large industry, make sure you are buying what is right for you. In the diet chapter, we suggested that you read labels to see what ingredients are in the foods that you eat. Do the same investigation with the cosmetics that you buy. Learn what it is that you are putting on your face and whether it is good for you.

We suggest that you stop buying cosmetics on impulse and buy only what suits your coloring. Once you have determined your look, buy into it. There are many looks to work toward in the years before "fiftysomething." Some women who have passed that mark, like actress Joan Collins, can still wear the darkest hair, the lightest skin, and the reddest lips. For others, a softer palette creates a quite different, yet equally attractive, face.

No amount of cosmetics can cover poorly cared-for skin. Begin cosmetic application with a clean face and a good moisturizer. We have a friend who prides herself on wearing only powder, light lipstick, and a touch of mascara most of the time, and she looks terrific. We have another who can't leave home without false eyelashes and a complete paint job. She looks good, too. They have chosen to make up in a way that makes them look and feel good. You choose for yourself what works for you. If you do choose a full range of makeup, be sure you know how to apply it artfully. Study yourself in daylight and in lamplight. The effects of your makeup change in different lights. You may find you need a lighter hand during the day.

However you feel about cosmetics and their use, if you use them, use them to your best advantage. That professional lesson we mentioned earlier can work wonders for you in helping you to pick your image and enhance it with makeup.

Dressing the Part

Hems go up and hems go down, but yours do not need to move, providing you have found a length the flatters you. Pants went in and out of fashion many times; today they seemed destined to be part of a woman's wardrobe forever. Now they simply swing from sleek to wide like a pendulum. All women like to adopt what is in style and to be fashionable, but if it isn't right for you, our best advice is don't do it.

We talked about choosing your role earlier in the book. Well, a role demands a few costume changes that, in every instance, complement the role. An artist dresses differently from an accountant; a homemaker dresses differently from a hard hat. In every case, it is important to determine what you want to look like and what flatters you. Have style; don't be trendy. Style can be defined as your look that never goes in or out of fashion; trend is what you learn is in or out and follow when you have not selected your own style.

A stylish woman, at midlife or at any time in life, makes a strong statement about herself. She defines how she sees herself and how she wishes to be seen. It works for her as long as she does not pick a style that is out of sync with her physical frame or her age. When we try to adopt an unflattering look, we will often be uncomfortable with it. So go to your closet. Put together all the clothes that you live in and put them on one end of the rod. Take all the things you bought that you never wear (excluding dressy things for rare occasions). The group of clothing that you wear all the time consists of those that help to define your role. Study them carefully. Take an extra minute to consider each piece and whether you like yourself in it. Then add to them or subtract from them according to wear and tear, but learn to know them as your comfort-level clothing. If you do, then they are your style. Now, study the group of seldom-worn clothes and realize your mistakes.

If you still feel confused, visit a department store and meet with the personal shopper. Most stores offer this valuable service at no charge, and you will probably find out a lot about what you like, what looks best on you, and what goes with what. Remember, too, that just as you may want to change your cosmetic color palette, or your hair color, you may also want to consider whether the colors that you choose in clothing are still the best colors for you.

Figuring out your style should be an enjoyable experience, and one that will add to your confidence when you are choosing what to buy or what to wear. If an outfit "isn't you," forget about buying it, because ultimately you will not wear it. Mostly, have fun deciding your role and costuming it.

Cosmetic Surgery

Cosmetic surgery, previously the domain of the rich and famous, has now become a standard option for millions of women. There are many ways to tuck, mold, fix, and shape faces and bodies. More and more young women are having eye lifts in their thirties and face-lifts in their forties than ever before. It is probably all part of the living longer, living better, looking better drive.

The five cosmetic surgery procedures performed most often are liposuction, which vacuums diet-resistant fat from young bodies; breast augmentation to add implants to bosoms; blepharoplasty, in which the upper eyelids lose their slouch and the lower ones lose their bags; face-lifts to turn the clock back ten years; and lip augmentation for all ages to enhance the thinning lips of age or to offer a model's pouty mouth.

If you are interested in knowing more about cosmetic surgery, choose a doctor very carefully and make a consultation appointment. The American Society of Plastic and Reconstructive Surgeons is listed in appendix D. The organization will provide names of surgeons and their credentials. Remember, it is good to see the results on several satisfied plastic surgery patients and to get a couple of opinions. Do not be afraid to ask questions. The only stupid question is the unasked one. Do not settle for a surgeon who is not interested in answering your questions, or in doing what you want to have done. Do not let a surgeon coerce you into unwanted procedures.

·12·

One, Two, Three—Go!

Your final step is to get going with the Utian Menopause Management Program. Starting is easy. Just check off the following ten steps to your personal success.

_____ 1. Review the Utian Menopause Management Program, chapter 2.

_____ 2. Schedule an appointment with your physician. List the questions you want to discuss in a format like the one we have provided on page 173.

_____ 3. Commit to changing your dietstyle; sign your contract in chapter 7, and don't break it!

_____ 4. Select your exercise program from chapter 8 and begin exercising.

_____ 5. Study yourself carefully and from all angles in a full-length mirror.

_____ 6. Determine the image you want to see, the role you want to play, and go for it.

_____ 7. Set up an appointment for a professional cosmetics consultation or begin to experiment yourself.

_____ 8. Examine your hair, nails, and skin and decide whether they need more help and care.

_____ 9. Tackle the clothes in your closet; separate those you wear from those you ignore.

_____10. Warn your family that you are about to get up and go!

As you go about the business of personal change, do not let anything or anyone dissuade you. Remember the underlying philosophy of our program: In the second half of your life, you owe it to yourself to do what you want to do. Good Luck!

Questions I Want to Ask My Doctor

1. _____
_____
_____
_____

2. _____
_____
_____
_____

3. _____
_____
_____
_____

4. _____
_____
_____
_____

5. _____
_____
_____
_____

6. _____
_____
_____
_____

Appendix A: Hormone Lists

Estrogens Available for Clinical Use

Natural Estrogens
The natural estrogens (called the conjugated estrogens by physicians because they have already been partially inactivated or softened) actually may be derived from natural or synthetic sources. They generally are more easily handled and excreted by the body. Your physician will select which one you should take. The group of natural estrogens include the following:

- Conjugated equine estrogens
- Esterified estrogens
- Estradiol-17β
- Estradiol cypionate
- Estradiol valerate
- Estrone and estrone sulfate
- Piperazine estrone sulfate
- Estradiol-17β micronized
- Polyestradiol phosphate
- Polyestriol phosphate
- Estriol succinate or hemisuccinate
- Estriol

Synthetic Steroids: Nonconjugated
The synthetic steroids, which are nonconjugated, represent the majority of oral contraceptives. These estrogens appear to affect various body processes such as levels of blood fats, lipoproteins, and choles-

terol differently than the so-called natural or conjugated estrogens. They also appear to have a greater effect on the enzyme processes of the liver (studies showed that ethinyl estradiol, a synthetic steroid, is about one hundred times as potent as equine estrogen, a natural one), so they are not popularly used in the United States for hormone replacement therapy.

There are three synthetic hormones:

- Ethinyl estradiol
- Methyl ethinyl estradiol (mestranol)
- Quinestrol

Synthetic Nonsteroids

This group includes diethylstilbestrol (DES), a drug used to avert threatened miscarriages in the 1950s, which achieved notoriety because it was linked to abnormalities in the daughters born to mothers who had taken this medication. Although the following group are potent estrogens, they are not popularly prescribed for hormone replacement therapy:

- Chlorotrianisene
- Dienestrol
- Diethylstilbestrol

The estrogens available for clinical use are listed in the following tables.

ORAL ESTROGENS

Estrogen	Trade Name	Pill Dose in mg	Pharmaceutical Co.
Ethinyl estradiol	Estinyl	0.02 0.05 0.5	Schering-Plough
Micronized estradiol	Estrace	1.0 2.0	Mead Johnson
Esterified Estrogens	Estratab	0.3 0.625 1.25 2.5	Reid-Rowell
Quinestrol	Estrovis	0.1	Parke-Davis
Estropipate (Piperazine estrone sulfate)	Ogen	0.625 1.25 2.5 5.0	Abbott
Conjugated estrogens	Premarin	0.3 0.625 0.9 1.25 2.5	Wyeth-Ayerst
Estradiol valerate	Progynova	1.0 2.0	Schering AG, Berlin

Source: Compiled by the author.

ESTROGEN VAGINAL CREAM

Generic Estrogen	Trade Name	Dose in mg/gm*	Pharmaceutical Co.
Diethylstilbestrol	Diethylstilbestrol suppositories	0.1 mg 0.5 mg	Lilly
Dienestrol	Estragard cream	0.01%	Reid-Rowell
Estradiol-17β	Estrace vaginal cream	0.1 mg	Mead Johnson
Estropipate	Ogen vaginal cream	1.5 mg	Abbott
Dienestrol	Ortho dienestrol cream	0.01%	Ortho
Conjugated estrogens	Premarin vaginal cream	0.625 mg	Wyeth-Ayerst

*Milligrams of drug per gram of cream.

PARENTERAL ESTROGENS

Generic Estrogen	Trade Name	Application Method	Dose	Pharmaceutical Company
Estradiol valerate	Delestrogen	Injection	10 mg 20 mg 40 mg	Squibb
Estradiol cypionate	Depo-Estradiol	Injection	1 mg 5 mg	Upjohn
Transdermal estradiol	Estraderm	Skin patch	0.05 mg/day 0.1 mg/day	Ciba-Geigy
Estradiol benzoate	Estradiol benzoate	Injection	0.5 mg/ml	Generic
Polyestradiol phosphate	Estradurin	Injection	40 mg/2 ml	Wyeth-Ayerst
Estradiol pellet	Estrapel*	Implant	25 mg	Bartor, Progynon
Estradiol valerate	Estraval	Injection	10 mg 20 mg	Reid-Rowell
Conjugated equine estrogen	Premarin IV	Injection	25 mg/ml	Wyeth-Ayerst
Estradiol-17β	Estrogel	Skin cream	3 mg	Key/LaSalle

*Temporarily suspended by FDA

179

Progesterone and Progestins (Progestogens)

There is only one natural progesterone. Until recently it could not be given by mouth and was thus given by intramuscular injection or vaginal suppositories. Neither of the latter are practical for HRT (see chapter 5). The orally active progesterone-like drugs are called progestins (progestogen). There are two types:

- Progesterone-like drugs derived from progesterone, for example, medroxyprogesterone acetate.
- Progesterone-like drugs derived from testosterone, for example, norethindrone, norgestrel.

PROGESTERONE AND PROGESTINS

Generic Name	Trade Name	Dose in mg	Pharmaceutical Co.
ORAL			
Medroxyprogesterone acetate	Amen	10	Carnick
Norethindrone acetate	Aygestin	5	Wyeth-Ayerst
Medroxyprogesterone acetate	Curretab	10	Reid-Rowell
Megestrol acetate	Megace	20	Bristol-Myers
		40	
Norethindrone	Micronor	0.35	Ortho
Norethindrone acetate	Norlutate	5	Parke-Davis
Norethindrone	Norlutin	5	Parke-Davis
Norethindrone	Nor-Q.D.	0.35	Syntex
Norgestrel	Ovrette	0.075	Wyeth-Ayerst
Medroxyprogesterone acetate	Provera	2.5	Upjohn
		5	
		10	
Micronized progesterone (capsule)	Uterogestin	150	Key/LaSalle
		300	
PROGESTERONE VAGINAL SUPPOSITORIES		25	Orphan Drug
		50	
		100	
		200	
INJECTABLE			
Medroxyprogesterone acetate	Depo-Provera	100, 400/ml	Upjohn

ANDROGENS

Generic Androgen	Trade Name	Dose	Pharmaceutical Co.
ORAL TABLETS			
Fluoxymesterone	Fluoxymesterone	5 mg	Reid-Rowell
Fluoxymesterone	Halotestin	5 mg	Upjohn
Methyltestosterone	Metandren	5 mg	Ciba-Geigy
Testosterone propionate	Oreton	5 mg	Schering
PARENTERAL			
Testosterone enanthate	Delatestryl	100 mg/ml	Squibb
Testosterone cypionate	Depo-Testosterone	50 mg/ml	Upjohn
Testosterone propionate	Oreton	75 mg	Schering
Testosterone pellets	Testopel	75 mg	Bartor
ESTROGEN/ANDROGEN COMBINATIONS			
Estradiol cypionate	Depo-Testadiol (injectable)	2 mg	Upjohn
Testosterone cypionate		50 mg	
Esterified estrogens	Estratest H.S. tablets	0.625 mg	Reid-Rowell
Methyl testosterone		1.25 mg	
Esterified estrogens	Estratest tablets	1.25 mg	Reid-Rowell
Methyl testosterone		2.5 mg	
Conjugated estrogens	Premarin with methyltestosterone	0.625 mg	Wyeth-Ayerst
Methyl testosterone		5 mg	
Conjugated estrogens	Premarin with methyltestosterone	1.25 mg	Wyeth-Ayerst
Methyl testosterone		10 mg	

Appendix B: Calcium, Fat, and Cholesterol Tables

Calcium

Current scientific recommendations for minimal daily calcium requirements are as follows:

Age	Milligrams Daily
Teenagers	1,200
Young adults	800–1,000
Women over 45	1,200–1,500

Ideally, this calcium should be obtained from a balanced diet. You could roughly estimate your calcium intake by listing your average daily food intake and then noting the calcium values from the following table. If your calcium intake is low, you could increase the amount by selectively increasing your intake of appropriate calcium-rich food items. If too many calories result, especially too much fat, calcium supplements may work for you. Some of the wide array of calcium supplements are listed in this appendix.

FOODS RICH IN CALCIUM—BUT WATCH THE FAT!

Serving Size	Food Item	Calcium (milligrams)	Fat (grams)
DAIRY PRODUCTS			
1 ounce	American cheese	200	8
1 ounce	Blue cheese	150	9
1 ounce	Cheddar cheese	200	9
1 cup	Cottage cheese	200	10
1 ounce	Mozzarella cheese	150	6
1 ounce	Swiss cheese	250	7
1 cup	Low-fat milk	300	5
1 cup	Skim milk	300	0.5
1 cup	Whole milk	300	8
1 cup	Yogurt (low-fat plain)	400	3
1 ounce	Ice cream, hard	200	14
FRUITS AND VEGETABLES			
5	Figs	125	1
1	Orange	50	
½ cup	Raisins	50	0.1
Small salad	Greens	100	
½ cup	Spinach, cooked	75	0.2
1 small	Sweet potato	50	0.5
1 ounce	Almonds, roasted	50	15
½ cup	Sunflower seeds	125	50
FISH			
3 ounces	Sardines	400	2
3 ounces	Scallops	110	1
3 ounces	Shrimp, raw	50	0.5
GENERAL			
1 ounce	Chocolate bar	64	9
1 slice of a 12-inch pizza	Pizza	150	5

Source: Compiled by the author.

CALCIUM SUPPLEMENTS

Calcium Type	Trade Name	Milligrams Calcium	Pharmaceutical Co.
Calcium lactate	Calcet	152.8	Mission
Calcium carbonate + vit. D	Caltrate 600 + Vit D	600 mg	Lederle
Calcium carbonate	Caltrate 600	600 mg	Lederle
Calcium carbonate + vit. D	Os-Cal 250	250 mg	Marion
Calcium carbonate	Os-Cal 500	500 mg	Marion
Calcium phosphate	Posture	600 mg	Ayerst
Calcium phosphate + vit. D	Posture with D	600 mg	Ayerst
Calcium carbonate	Tums	200 mg	Norcliff-Thayer
Calcium citrate	Citracal	100 mg	Mission

Source: Compiled by the author.
Note: Calcium carbonate provides approximately 40 percent elemental calcium by weight; lactate, phosphate and citrate about 20 percent elemental calcium.

Fat

Fat should not comprise more than 30 percent of your daily calories. Thus, a 2,000-calorie diet would allow you about 67 grams of fat. Remember that fats are high in calories. Saturated fats, usually present in roasted, fried, baked, or broiled foods, are to be avoided.

The table below should act as a guide to reducing high-fat, high-calorie foods. The source of information is the Human Nutrition Information Service, U.S. Department of Agriculture. For comprehensive fat and calorie values for many other foods, consider purchasing *Nutritive Value of Foods,* HG-72, available from the Superintendent of Documents, U.S. Government Printing Office, Washington, D.C. 20402.

Evidence is increasing that eating too much fat (both saturated and unsaturated) may increase your risk of suffering cancer of the colon, breast, prostate, or uterus (endometrium). A good resource on dietary fat and fiber is published by the U.S. Department of Health and Human Services, NIH Publication No. 85-2711, entitled *Diet, Nutrition and Cancer Prevention.*

FAT/CALORIE CHART

Food	Serving	Calories	Grams of Fat
DAIRY PRODUCTS			
Cheese			
American, pasteurized process	1 oz	105	9
Cheddar	1 oz	115	9
Cottage			
Creamed	½ cup	115	5
Low-fat (2%)	½ cup	100	2
Cream	1 oz	100	10
Mozzarella, part skim	1 oz	80	5
Parmesan	1 tbsp	25	2
Swiss	1 oz	105	8
Cream			
Half and half	2 tbsp	40	3
Light, coffee, or table	2 tbsp	60	6
Sour	2 tbsp	50	5
Ice Cream	1 cup	270	14

FAT/CALORIE CHART *(continued)*

Food	Serving	Calories	Grams of Fat
Ice Milk	1 cup	185	6
Milk			
Whole	1 cup	150	8
Low-fat (2%)	1 cup	125	5
Nonfat, skim	1 cup	85	trace
Yogurt, low-fat, fruit-flavored	8 oz	230	2
MEATS			
Beef, cooked			
Braised or pot-roasted			
Less lean cuts, such as chuck blade, lean only	3 oz	255	16
Leaner cuts, such as bottom round, lean only	3 oz	190	8
Ground beef, broiled			
Lean	3 oz	230	15
Regular	3 oz	245	17
Roast, oven cooked			
Less lean cuts, such as rib, lean only	3 oz	225	15
Leaner cuts, such as eye of round, lean only	3 oz	155	6
Steak, sirloin, broiled			
Lean and fat	3 oz.	250	17
Lean only	3 oz	185	8
Lamb, cooked			
Chops, loin, broiled			
Lean and fat	3 oz	250	17
Lean only	3 oz	185	8
Leg, roasted, lean only	3 oz	160	7
Pork, cured, cooked			
Bacon, fried	3 slices	110	9
Ham, roasted			
Lean and fat	3 oz	205	14
Lean only	3 oz	135	5
Pork, fresh, cooked			
Chop, center loin			
Broiled			
Lean and fat	3 oz	270	19
Lean only	3 oz	195	9

FAT/CALORIE CHART *(continued)*

Food	Serving	Calories	Grams of Fat
Pan-fried			
Lean and fat	3 oz	320	26
Lean only	3 oz	225	14
Rib, roasted, lean only	3 oz	210	12
Shoulder, braised, lean only	3 oz	210	10
Spareribs, braised, lean and fat	3 oz	340	26
Veal cutlet, braised or broiled	3 oz	185	9
Sausages			
Bologna	2 oz	180	16
Frankfurters	2 oz (1 frank)	185	17
Pork, link or patty, cooked	2 oz (4 links)	210	18
Salami, cooked type	2 oz	145	11
POULTRY PRODUCTS			
Chicken, fried, flour-coated			
Dark meat with skin	3 oz	240	14
Light meat with skin	3 oz	210	10
Chicken, roasted			
Dark meat without skin	3 oz	175	8
Light meat without skin	3 oz	145	4
Duck, roasted, meat			
without skin	3 oz	170	10
Turkey, roasted			
Dark meat without skin	3 oz	160	6
Light meat without skin	3 oz	135	3
Egg, hard cooked	1 large	80	6
SEAFOOD			
Flounder, baked			
With butter or margarine	3 oz	120	6
Without butter or margarine	3 oz	85	1
Oysters, raw	3 oz	55	2
Shrimp, French fried	3 oz	200	10
Shrimp, boiled or steamed	3 oz	100	1
Tuna, packed in oil, drained	3 oz	165	7
Tuna, packed in water, drained	3 oz	135	1

FAT/CALORIE CHART *(continued)*

Food	Serving	Calories	Grams of Fat
GRAIN PRODUCTS			
Bread, white	1 slice	65	1
Biscuit, 2½ inches across	one	135	5
Muffin, plain, 2½ inches across	one	120	4
Pancake, 4 inches across	one	60	2
OTHER FOODS			
Avocado	½	160	15
Butter, margarine	1 tbsp	100	12
Cake, white layer, chocolate frosting	1 piece	265	11
Cookies, chocolate chip	4	185	11
Donut, yeast type, glazed	one	235	13
Mayonnaise	1 tbsp	100	11
Oils	1 tbsp	120	14
Peanut butter	1 tbsp	95	8
Peanuts	½ cup	420	35
Salad dressing			
Regular	1 tbsp	65	6
Low-calorie	1 tbsp	20	1

Source: Compiled from the *Human Nutrition Information Service,* U.S. Department of Agriculture.

Cholesterol-Rich Foods

Cholesterol is a necessary component of body function, with usually about one-third coming from the average diet and two-thirds being produced by the body itself. An increase in dietary cholesterol increases the levels of cholesterol in the blood, which may heighten your risk of heart attack.

Avoidance of cholesterol-rich foods should be considered carefully in planning your own diet. If you have an elevated blood cholesterol level (see chapter 7), then reducing your intake of these foods is a first step toward reducing your risk of heart disease.

Usually, fruits and vegetables do not contain any cholesterol. Some higher-carbohydrate foods like noodles, spaghetti, white bread, or cornbread are very low in cholesterol.

Food Item	Serving Size	Cholesterol (Milligrams)
DAIRY PRODUCTS		
Cheese		
American, pasteurized	1 ounce	30
Cheddar	1 ounce	30
Cottage, creamed	1 ounce	34
Cottage, low-fat 2%	1 ounce	20
Swiss	1 ounce	28
Milk		
Whole	1 cup	33
Buttermilk	1 cup	10
Cream	½ cup	40
Low-fat 2%	1 cup	18
Skim	1 cup	4
Yogurt		
Low-fat	1 cup	15
Regular	1 cup	30
MEATS		
Beef	3 ounces	80
Lamb	3 ounces	83
Liver	3 ounces	350
Pork	3 ounces	75
Veal	3 ounces	85
POULTRY PRODUCTS		
Chicken	3 ounces	40–60
Chicken noodle soup	1 cup	6
Chicken chow mein	3 ounces	45
Egg	1 large	270
Turkey pie	3 ounces	80
SEAFOOD		
Fish fillet	3 ounces	40–80
Clams	3 ounces	50

Food Item	Serving Size	Cholesterol (Milligrams)
Lobster	3 ounces	75
Oysters	3 ounces	40
Shrimp	3 ounces	130

GRAIN GROUP
All essentially low except egg noodles.

DESSERTS
Custard	½ cup	140
Lemon meringue pie	14 ounces	100
Ice cream	½ cup	40
Lady fingers	4	160

Source: Compiled by the author.

Appendix C: Metropolitan Height and Weight Tables

To Make an Approximation of Your Frame Size . . .

Extend your arm and bend the forearm upward at a ninety-degree angle. Keep fingers straight and turn the inside of your wrist toward your body. If you have a caliper, use it to measure the space between the two prominent bones on either side of your elbow. Without a caliper, place thumb and index finger of your other hand on these two bones. Measure the space between your fingers against a ruler or tape measure. Compare it with these tables that list elbow measurements for medium-framed men and women. Measurements lower than those listed indicate you have a small frame. Higher measurements indicate a large frame.

Height in 1" heels	Elbow Breadth	Height in 1" heels	Elbow Breadth
MEN		WOMEN	
5'2"–5'3"	2½"–2⅞"	4'10"–4'11"	2¼"–2½"
5'4"–5'7"	2⅝"–2⅞"	5'0"–5'3"	2¼"–2½"
5'8"–5'11"	2¾"–3"	5'4"–5'7"	2⅜"–2⅝"
6'0"–6'3"	2¾"–3⅛"	5'8"–5'11"	2⅜"–2⅝"
6'4"	2⅞"–3¼"	6'0"	2½"–2¾"

1983 METROPOLITAN HEIGHT AND WEIGHT TABLES

WOMEN

Height Feet	Inches	Small Frame	Medium Frame	Large Frame
4	10	102–111	109–121	118–131
4	11	103–113	111–123	120–134
5	0	104–115	113–126	122–137
5	1	106–118	115–129	125–140
5	2	108–121	118–132	128–143
5	3	111–124	121–135	131–147
5	4	114–127	124–138	134–151
5	5	117–130	127–141	137–155
5	6	120–133	130–144	140–159
5	7	123–136	133–147	143–163
5	8	126–139	136–150	146–167
5	9	129–142	139–153	149–170
5	10	132–145	142–156	152–173
5	11	135–148	145–159	155–176
6	0	138–151	148–162	158–179

MEN

Height Feet	Inches	Small Frame	Medium Frame	Large Frame
5	2	128–134	131–141	138–150
5	3	130–136	133–143	140–153
5	4	132–138	135–145	142–156
5	5	134–140	137–148	144–160
5	6	136–142	139–151	146–164
5	7	138–145	142–154	149–168
5	8	140–148	145–157	152–172
5	9	142–151	148–160	155–176
5	10	144–154	151–163	158–180
5	11	146–157	154–166	161–184
6	0	149–160	157–170	164–188
6	1	152–164	160–174	168–192
6	2	155–168	164–178	172–197
6	3	158–172	167–182	176–202
6	4	162–176	171–187	181–207

Source: Courtesy of Metropolitan Life Insurance Company.

Appendix D: Resources for Seeking Information or Help

OSTEOPOROSIS
National Osteoporosis Foundation
1625 Eye Street, N.W., No. 822
Washington, DC 20006
(202) 223-2226
(Information on osteoporosis)

MENOPAUSE RESOURCES
International Menopause Society
8 avenue Don Bosco
1150 Brussels
Belgium
(An excellent resource for
  addresses of national menopause
  societies)

North American Menopause
  Society
c/o Cleveland Menopause Clinic
29001 Cedar Road, No. 600
Cleveland, OH 44124
(Information on menopause, lists
  of known menopause centers)

GENERAL
American Association of Retired
  Persons
1909 K Street, N.W.
Washington, DC 20049
(202) 728-4450

D.E.S. Action National

East Coast Office:
  Long Island Jewish-Hillside
    Medical Center
  New Hyde Park
  New York, NY 11040
  (516) 775-3450

West Coast Office:
  2845 24th Street
  San Francisco, CA 94110
  (415) 826-5060
(Provides medical information and
  physician referral to women
  given DES during pregnancy
  [1941–1971] and to their
  daughters and sons)

Endometriosis Association
  Headquarters
8585 N. 76th Place
Milwaukee, WI 53203
(800) 992-ENDO (United States)
(800) 426-2 END (Canada)
(Provides support, education, and
  research on all aspects of
  endometriosis)

MEDICAL ORGANIZATIONS
American Academy of Family
   Physicians
8880 W. Parkway
Kansas City, MO 64114
(800) 274-2237

American College of Obstetricians
   and Gynecologists
Attn: Resource Center
409 12th Street S.W.
Washington, DC 20024-2188
(202) 638-5577

American College of Physicians
Independence Mall West, Sixth
   Street at Race
Philadelphia, PA 19106

American Fertility Society
1608 13th Avenue South, No. 101
Birmingham, AL 35256
(205) 933-8494

American Society of Plastic
   & Reconstructive Surgeons
   (ASPRS)
233 N. Michigan Avenue, No.
   1900
Chicago, IL 60601

DENTAL
American Dental Association
211 E. Chicago Avenue
Chicago, IL 60611

Appendix E: Useful Reading and Resource Material

MEDICAL BOOKS

Exercise Testing and Training of Apparently Healthy Individuals by the Committee on Exercise of the American Heart Association (American Heart Association, 1972).

Another resource manual for physicians on techniques of exercise testing and appropriate training.

Guidelines for Exercise Testing and Prescription by American College of Sports Medicine (Lea and Febiger, Philadelphia, Third Edition, 1986).

This is *the* resource manual for techniques of exercise testing.

Menopause in Modern Perspective by Wulf H. Utian, M.D., Ph.D. (Appleton, New York, 1980).

A comprehensive monograph for practicing physicians.

Menopause—Physiology and Pharmacology edited by Daniel R. Mishell (Year Book Medical Publishers, Chicago, 1987).

A detailed review with contributions by thirty-seven authors directed essentially at medical scientists and practitioners.

The Menopause edited by John Studd and Malcolm Whitehead (Blackwell, Boston, 1988).

A review by twenty-eight international contributors aimed at physicians and medical scientists.

The Social and Psychological Origins of the Climacteric Syndrome by John Gerald Greene (Gower, Aldershot, UK, 1984).

An elucidating review of psychosocial aspects as researched by nurses, sociologists, psychologists, psychiatrists, gynecologists, and anthropologists.

GENERAL BOOKS

Beauty Bound by Rita Freedman, Ph.D. (D.C. Heath, New York, 1986).
Describes how body image affects mental health and gives recommendations on enhancing self-image through cosmetic surgery.

Controlling Cholesterol by Kenneth H. Cooper (Bantam Books, New York, 1988).
One of the best of the many books written on techniques for reducing cholesterol and preventing heart attacks.

Endometriosis by Julia Older (Charles Scribner's Sons, New York, 1984).
An excellent overview of endometriosis, its diagnosis, and treatment.

Estrogen—The Facts Can Change Your Life by Lila Nachtigall, M.D. and Joan Rattner Heilman (Harper & Row, New York, 1986).
Descriptions of estrogen replacement therapy and ways to take it.

How a Woman Ages by Robin Marantz Henig (Ballantine Books, New York, 1985).
Describes the processes of growing older and what you can do about it.

How to Avoid a Hysterectomy by Lynn Payer (Pantheon Books, New York, 1987).
A short, well-written guide to exploring all options before consenting to a hysterectomy.

Hysterectomy: Before and After by Winnifred B. Cutler (Harper & Row, New York, 1988).
A comprehensive guide to preventing or preparing for, and managing health after, hysterectomy.

Love, Sex, and Aging by Edward M. Brecher (Consumers Union, Mount Vernon, NY, 1984).
A Consumer Union report into the love and sex lives of the older person. Revealing and encouraging.

Once a Month: A Guide to the Effects, Diagnosis and Treatment of Premenstrual Syndrome by Katharina Dalton, M.D. (Hunter House, Claremont, CA, 1986).
The first physician to describe the use of natural progesterone for PMS, as of yet still a controversial treatment.

Osteoporosis—The Silent Thief by William A. Peck, M.D. and Louis V. Avioli, M.D. (AARP Books, Glenview, IL, 1988).
A very readable and balanced explanation of osteoporosis causes, diagnosis, risks, prevention, and treatment.

Ourselves Growing Older by Paula Brown Doress and Diana Laskin Siegal (Simon and Schuster, New York, 1987).

> Written in cooperation with the Boston Women's Health Book Collective, this book reviews aging in women, coping techniques, and enhancement of self-power.

Royal Canadian Air Force Exercise Plans for Physical Fitness by R.C.A.F. (Pocket Books, New York, 1972).

> Still the classic balanced exercise program demanding less than twenty minutes per day of your time.

Safe Encounters by Beverly Whipple and Gina Ogden (McGraw-Hill, New York, 1989).

> An attempt to describe safer sex techniques while conscious of the fear of AIDS and other sexually transmitted diseases.

Save Your Money, Save Your Face by Elaine Brumberg (Harper & Row, New York, 1986).

> Described as the Ralph Nader of the cosmetics industry, essential information is provided on cosmetics, skin care products, and skin care.

The New Our Bodies, Ourselves by the Boston Women's Health Book Collective (Simon and Schuster, New York, 1985).

> An overview of a full spectrum of women's health issues.

The Seasons of a Man's Life by Daniel J. Levinson (Alfred A. Knopf, New York, 1978).

> An excellent resource on male behavior indicating how every grown man passes through a series of age-linked phases that underlie his personal crises.

Your Skin from Acne to Zits by Jerome Z. Litt, M.D. (Dembner Books, New York, 1989).

> A leading dermatologist helps you treat dozens of common skin ailments with over-the-counter remedies.

Appendix F: Ask the Doctor

Twenty of the Most Frequently Asked Questions in the Office and at Medical Seminars

Q. What are the risks of pregnancy at the "change-of-life" period?

A. There is always a chance of pregnancy as long as you are menstruating. Toward the end of the reproductive years some cycles are non-egg-producing, but you should not rely on this fact. Always use appropriate contraception.

Q. I had my uterus and cervix removed. Should I still get a PAP test, and how often?

A. The vaginal PAP test is still useful as a hormonal test. There are changes in the vaginal cells that indicate whether you are losing estrogen, so the test continues to have a medical benefit.

Q. Does someone who has had a hysterectomy go through menopause at an earlier age?

A. Probably not. There are some women who have an abnormal blood supply to their ovaries and the surgery might be disruptive. In that instance, an early menopause can occur.

Q. If I had a hysterectomy, how will I know that I have become menopausal?

A. You will either develop symptoms like hot flashes, sleep disturbances, and vaginal discomfort, or you could have a blood test to measure the FSH level. Elevation of the latter indicates that you are into menopause.

Q. I am forty-one years old and have been experiencing changes in my body for the past three years. Why don't the doctors listen more to what I say rather than to what my age is?

A. Menopause can occur earlier, and the symptoms are variable. Ask your doctor the question directly. If you do not get satisfactory answers, seek help elsewhere.

Q. How often should I have mammograms after age fifty, especially if there is a family history of breast cancer?

A. We recommend that all women have mammograms every two years from ages forty to fifty and annually after age fifty. If on hormone therapy, it is advisable to have a twice-yearly breast examination.

Q. Is there a risk in having a bone scan?

A. The amount of x-ray in a bone scan is extremely small, and certainly not more than the scatter you would be exposed to on an airplane flight from Los Angeles to New York.

Q. Does the presence of fibroid tumors inside the uterus necessitate a hysterectomy prior to hormone replacement therapy?

A. No. The fibroids should be treated according to the usual accepted general principles. If they of themselves require surgery, then it is best undertaken before starting hormone replacement therapy. HRT can cause the fibroids to increase in size and could lead to the need for a hysterectomy at a later date.

Q. Does HRT prevent weight loss?

A. There is minimal weight gain on HRT. Unless otherwise counseled by your doctor, you should incorporate the healthy diet and exercise program outlined in chapters 7 and 8 when commencing HRT.

Q. Is it true that estrogen can cause blood clotting?

A. There is little evidence. The early high-dose oral contraceptives did cause this problem, but the usual type of estrogen and progestin used after the menopause does not have the same effect.

Q. I have become more emotional and irritable since starting on HRT. Is this normal, and will it ever end?

A. It is not a normal response to HRT. You should discuss the type of hormones and the dosage with your physician. In particular, the progestin might be causing a problem.

Q. How long does one stay on estrogen therapy?

A. As long as you feel good and believe you are achieving benefits from the treatment. Many women will remain on therapy for ten, fifteen, or even twenty years.

Q. Is there any help for a woman who can't tolerate progestin?

A. It is possible that the estrogen could be given alone, but the uterine lining should be sampled (biopsied) at least once yearly to be certain that no abnormal responses are occurring.

Q. I am sixty-seven years old. I had a natural menopause and have all my parts. Is it too late to take estrogen?

A. No, it is never too late. However, as for all women, there should be medical indication for starting treatment. You should not take it simply because your best friend does.

Q. If I was unable to take the birth control pill due to migraines, will I be able to consider HRT once my ovaries stop functioning?

A. Menstrual or birth control pill migraines are well-recognized problems that are difficult to treat. Fortunately, the hormones you take after menopause are weaker than those used in the birth control pill, and migraine is not usually a problem.

Q. I had an early menopause before age forty and am now fifty-one. What has my body lost in these eleven years, and what can I hope to regain?

A. You may have suffered bone loss, which could be confirmed by densitometry. A small percentage of this loss can be regained and further loss can be prevented. Tissues like the vaginal lining and skin can be considerably enhanced by starting HRT.

Q. Ten years ago I had breast cancer. Can I take estrogen therapy?

A. There is currently little evidence about the recurrence of breast cancer when HRT is given. Physicians are hesitant to prescribe under these circumstances and women are hesitant to take HRT. The general consensus is that women with previous breast cancer should not take these hormones.

Q. What should I believe about the risk of HRT and breast cancer in light of recent magazine and newspaper articles?

A. There are some indications that the risk of breast cancer might be increased by prolonged exposure to estrogen therapy. There is also no evidence to suggest that progestin will protect against the slight increase in risk. The level of increased risk is from about one case per thousand per year to between 1.2 and 1.9 cases per thousand per year after a minimum of six to nine years of hormone therapy. Most of the data has been related to the use of ethinyl estradiol, which is a potent estrogen not normally used in the United States for postmenopausal treatment. One reassuring factor has been the fact that the mortality rates for breast cancer in the United States have not increased over the last decade. However, anyone contemplating HRT should have a full checkup including mammography and repeated examinations as long as they remain on HRT. Indeed, they should be examined even if they are not on HRT.

Q. I dislike the return of my menstrual period on HRT. Will I have to suffer this as long as I am on HRT?

A. With cyclic HRT, over two-thirds of women have a menstrual period. But the cyclic therapy is the type proven to have the best benefits. Combined continuous hormones may avoid bleeding, but the outcome in terms of prevention of bone loss and heart disease and risk for breast cancer is still unknown. The bleeding is probably the single biggest nuisance factor you will have to tolerate in exchange for the benefits. As time goes by, the bleeding often lessens or even stops completely.

Q. Do family doctors have this updated information? Should premenopausal women see a specialist to be put on HRT?

A. Information regarding menopause and the use of postmenopausal hormones has escalated in the last several years. You should feel comfortable asking your family practitioner, internist, or gynecologist whether they are knowledgeable in the subject and would supervise your care, but it's always fine to obtain a second opinion if you would feel better having it.

Notes

Chapter 1: Living Longer, Living Better

6   Robert A. Wilson, *Feminine Forever* (New York: Mayflower-Dell, 1966).

8   "Fat women lose their periods": Statement attributed to Aetios of Amida, a prominent sixth-century A.D. writer. d.V. Ricci, trans., *Cornarius* (Philadelphia: Blakeston, 1950).

8   John Leake, *Chronic or Slow Diseases Peculiar to Women* (London: Baldwin, 1777).

9   "A lady who has during": H. Charrasse, *Advice to a Wife* (Philadelphia: Lippincott, 1868).

9   "Compelled to yield to the power": Columbat de L'Isere, *Treatise on the Diseases of Females,* trans. C. D. Meigs and L. Blanchard (Philadelphia: Lea, 1845).

10 "A large percentage of women": R. A. Wilson and T. A. Wilson, "The Fate of the Nontreated Postmenopausal," *American Geriatric Society Journal* 11:347, 1963.

Chapter 3: Finding Dr. Right

21 Results of a 1970 European Menopause and Midlife Survey, International Health Foundation, Geneva, Switzerland.

21 Results of a 1987 Louis Harris Internal Medical Survey, Louis Harris Associates, London and New York.

38–39 Findings of a National Institutes of Health study. J. Perlman, P. Wolf, F. Finucane, and I. Madans, "Menopause and the Epidemiology of Cardiovascular Disease in Women," *Progress in Clinical and Biological Research,* 320, 283–312, 1989.

41 Findings of the Framingham Study, William B. Kannel and Tavia Gordon. Daniel R. Mishell, Jr., ed., "Cardiovascular Effects of the Menopause," *Menopause, Physiology, and Pharmacology,* 91–102. (Chicago: Yearbook Medical Publishers, 1987).

41   Results of a study conducted by Ronald Ross. England, *Lancet* 1, 858, 1981.

41   Findings of a Boston study. M. J. Stampfer, W. C. Willett, J. A. Colditz, et al., "A Prospective Study of Postmenopausal Estrogen Therapy and Coronary Heart Disease," *New England Journal of Medicine,* 313: 1044.

45   Findings of a Framingham study, 18-year follow up. William B. Kannel and Tavia Gordon, eds., The Framingham Study, section 30, Washington DC, Department of Health Education, and Welfare Publication, 74-599, 1974.

45   Findings of a Scandinavian study. B. Procope, "Studies on the Urinary Excretion, Biological Effects and Origin of Oesthogens in Post-menopausal Women," *Acta Endocrinology* Supplement 135:1, 1968.

46   "The reasons often cited for removing healthy ovaries": W. H. Utian, *Menopause in Modern Perspective* (New York: ACC, 1980).

47   Findings of a Boston Collaborative Drug Surveillance Program analysis. H. Jick, J. Porter, and A. S. Morrison, "Relationship Between Smoking and the Age of Natural Menopause," *Lancet* 1:1354, 1977.

Chapter 4: Your Helpful Early-Warning System

56   Katherina Dalton, *The Premenstrual Syndrome and Progesterone Therapy* (London: Heinemann, 1977).

Chapter 5: Taking Control of Your Own Life

65   "[Brown-Sequard] wrote that he achieved greater body vigor": d.V. Ricci, *One Hundred Years of Gynecology, 1800–1900* (Philadelphia: Blakeston, 1945).

66   A. S. Parkes and C. W. Bellerby, "Studies on the Internal Secretions of the Ovary" and "The Distribution in the Ovary of the Oestrus-Producing Hormone," *Journal of Physiology* 61:563, 1926.

66   A. Butenandt, Uber die Reindarstellung des Follikel-hormons aus Schwangerenharn, *ZF Physiology Chem* 191:127, 1930.

74   "The combined continuous method attempts to avoid . . . withdrawal bleeding": G. Culberg, F. Knutsson, L. A. Mattson, "A New Combination of Conjugated Equine Oestrogens and Medroxyprogesterone for Treatment of Climacteric Complaints," *Maturitas* 61:55, 1984; and L. A. Mattson, G. Culberg, G. Samsoe, "Evaluation of a Continuous Oestrogen-Progesterone Regimen for Climacteric Complaints," *Maturitas* 4:95, 1982.

81   "Estrogen therapy offered an enhanced feeling of general well-being"—W. H. Utian, "The Mental Tonic Effect of Oestrogens Administered to Oophorectomized Females," *South African Medical Journal* 46:1079, 1972.

Chapter 6: Choices and Chances: Are Hormone Treatments Right for You?

88   "These potent hormones should ideally not": W. H. Utian, "Feminine Forever? Current Concepts on the Menopause. A Critical Review," *South African Journal of Obstetrics and Gynecology* 6:7–10, 1968.

88–   D. C. Smith, R. Prentice, DJ Thomson, and W. Herrman, "Associa-
89   tion of Exogenous Estrogen and Endometrial Carcinoma," *New England Journal of Medicine* 293:1164, 1975; and H. K. Ziel and W. D. Finkle, "Increased Risk of Endometrial Carcinoma Among Users of Conjugated Estrogens," *New England Journal of Medicine* 293:1167, 1975.

91   "Studies of blood-clotting factors": R. J. Chetkowski, D. R. Meldrum, and K. A. Steingold, "Biologic Effects of Transdermal Estradiol," *New England Journal of Medicine* 314: 1615–1620, 1986.

93–   "Women who had lost ovarian function": W. H. Utian, "The Mental
94   Tonic Effect of Oestrogens Administered to Oophorectomized Females," *South African Medical Journal* 468:1079, 1972.

94   Findings of Harvard studies. I. Schiff, Q. Regestein Tulchinsky, and K. J. Ryan, "Effects of Estrogens on Sleep and the Psychological State of Hypo-gonadal Women," *Journal American Medical Association* 242: 2405–2407, 1979.

94   Findings of a King's College Hospital study. S. Campbell, "Double-blind Psychometric Studies on the Effects of Natural Oestrogens in Postmenopausal Women," *The Management of Menopause and Post-menopausal Years*, ed. S. Campbell (Lancaster: MTP Press, 1976).

97   Findings of a study by ten North American Lipid Research Clinics. T. L. Bush and E. Barrett-Connar, "Non-Contraceptive Estrogen Use and Cardiovascular Disease," *Epidemiology Review* 7:80, 80–99, 1985; and T. L. Bush, E. Barrett-Connar, and L. D. Cowan, "Cardiovascular Mortality and Non-Contraceptive Use of Estrogen in Women: Results from the Lipid Research Clinics Program Follow-up Study," *Circulation 75*, 1102, 1987.

Chapter 8: Getting Physical: Exercise and Sports

118   "Most studies show that mood-enhancing": R. S. Serfass, "Exercise for the Elderly—What are the Benefits and How do we get Started?" eds. E. L. Smith and R. S. Serfass, *Exercise and Aging* (Hillside, N. J.: Enslow, 121–9, 1981; and W. W. Sperduso, "Exercise as a Factor in Aging Motor Behavior Plasticity," *Exercise and Health,* American Academy of Physical Education Papers (Champaign, IL: Human Kinetics Publishers, 89–100, 1984).

118   Studies on weight-bearing exercises. B. L. Drinkwater, "Exercise and the Postmenopausal Woman," *Proceedings of the Fourth International*

Congress on the Menopause, ed. P. Van Keep, (Boston: MTP Press, 41–48, 1986). B. Krolner, B. Taft, S. P. Nelson, et al., "Physical Exercise as Prophylaxis against Involutional Bone Loss: A Controlled Trial," *Clinical Science* 64:541–546, 1983. J. F. Aloia, S. H. Cohn, T. Babu, et al, "Skeletal Mass and Body Composition in Marathon Runners," *Metabolism* 27:1793–1796, 1978. E. L. Smith, W. Reddan, and P. E. Smith, "Physical Activity and Calcium Modalities for Bone Mineral Increase in Aged Women," *Medical Science Sports Exercise* 13:60–64, 1981. M. K. Leere Koper, K. Tolia, and A. M. Parfitt, "Nutritional Endocrine and Demographic Aspects of Osteoporosis," *Orthopedics Clinical, North America* 12:547–558, 1981. J. F. Aloia, S. H. Cohn, J. A. Ostune, et al, "Prevention of Involutional Bone Loss by Exercise," *Annals of Internal Medicine* 89:356–358, 1978.

Chapter 9: Good, Better, Best: Sexuality and Aging

137   "Compelled to yield to the power": Colombat de L'Isere, *Treatise on the Diseases of Females,* trans. C. D. Meigs and L. Blanchard (Philadelphia: Lea, 1845).

138   Alfred Kinsey, *Sexual Behavior in the Human Female* (Philadelphia: Saunders, 1953).

138   William Masters and Virginia Johnson, *Human Sexual Response* (Boston: Little, Brown, 1966).

140   "As your estrogen level increases, your ability to discriminate": Personal communication between the author and Sarrel P.

145   Report from the Harvard Nurses Health Study. I. Comiev, W. C. Willett, G. A. Colditz, M. J. Stampfer, B. Rosner, C. H. Hennekens, and F. E. Speizer, "Prospective Study of Oral Contraceptive Use and Risk of Breast Cancer in Women," *Journal of the National Cancer Institute* 81:17, 1989.

150   "Specific instructions and techniques for masturbation": L. G. Barbach, *For Yourself: The Fulfillment of Female Sexuality* (New York, Anchor/Doubleday, 1976); and Stephen B. Levine, *Sex Is Not Simple* (Ohio: Ohio Publishing Co., 1988).

153   "Women of advanced maternal age delivering": W. H. Utian and R. Kiwi, "Obstetrical Risks of Pregnancy and Childbirth After Age 35," *Maturitas,* suppl. 63–72, 1988.

Chapter 10: Men and Menopause

156   "There are minor chemical changes": N. Kies, "Die Klimakterische Symptomatologie aus Klinisch-Psychologischer Sicht, *Med. Welt* 25: 228, 1974.

Glossary

absorptiometry—see bone densitometry
acute—sudden onset; opposite of chronic
administer—to give treatment
aerobic capacity—the amount of air breathed in a given time
alleviate—make less, improve or cure
amenorrhea—disappearance of menstrual periods
anatomy—description of body parts and structures
androgens—hormones with male-like effects
anemia—reduced amount of red blood cells
antidepressants—mood-elevating medications
anus—the opening of the lower bowel to the outside
anxiety—worrying without having something to worry about
artery—the blood vessels that leave the heart and carry blood to the rest of the body
arthritis—inflammation of joint(s)
atheromatosis—fatty disease of the blood vessels
atherosclerosis—hardening of the arteries
atrophic vaginitis thinning and inflammation of the vagina
atrophy—shrinking, reduction in size
Bartholin's gland—two glands at the entrance of the vagina that respond to sexual arousal by producing lubricating mucus
biofeedback—technique of controlling involuntary body functions by mind or conscious control
birth control pill—the oral contraceptive; a combination of estrogen and progestin in a pill that prevents ovulation and pregnancy
bladder—the storage bag in which urine collects before it is released
blood clot—a congealed lump of blood inside the blood vessel
blood stream—the rivers of blood inside the blood vessel
blood vessels—the tubes called arteries or veins in which blood flows

bone densitometry—a test to measure the amount (density) of bone

brain—the gray mass of nervous tissue inside the skull

breakthrough bleeding—vaginal bleeding that actually starts while taking female hormones or oral contraceptives

breast—milk-producing gland

calcium—the major chemical substance needed to harden bones and teeth

calories—essentially a measure of how much energy is present in the food one eats

cancer—uncontrolled growth of abnormal tissue that spreads and destroys normal tissue

carcinoma—see cancer

castration—removal of a woman's ovaries or a man's testicles

cell—the basic unit or building block out of which all body tissues are constructed

cervix—the mouth of the womb; the entrance of the uterus

change of life—see climacteric

cholesterol—an essential steroid chemical; excess implicated with heart disease

chronic—present or developing over a long period of time; opposite of acute

climacteric—the transition from reproductive to postreproductive age

climacteric syndrome—symptoms associated with the climacteric

clitoris—a small structure near the entrance of the vulva that is responsive to sexual stimulation

complaint—a symptom bad enough to bother the patient and to report to the doctor

complication—an adverse effect; development of one disease upon another

compression fracture—a weakened bone that cannot support weight and can break by being crushed

computerized axial tomography (CAT scan)—multiple x-ray technique for body imaging in disease diagnosis

condom—rubber sheath worn over penis

congenital—occurring from birth but not inherited

conjugated estrogen—a partially metabolized estrogen

contraceptive—technique for preventing pregnancy

contraindication—circumstances in which a drug should not be prescribed

Cooper's ligament—fibrous breast-supporting ligament

coronary artery disease—fatty disease of the arteries of the heart that can lead to plugging with a blood clot; see atheromatosis

corpus luteum—the yellow body in the ovary that forms from graafian follicle after ovulation

corticosteroids/cortisol—the cortisone group of steroids

culture—the usual beliefs, social behavior, and material components of a racial, religious, or social group, normally passed from one generation to the next

cycle—a recurring series of events; moving in a circle

cyclic regimen—interrupted episodes with ongoing medication

cyclical—used to refer to medical treatment of a regular but recurring on-off-on schedule

cytotoxic agent—chemical drugs poisonous to certain cells, for example, cancer

D & C—dilatation and curettage; common gynecologic operation in which the cervix is opened or stretched (dilatation), and the lining of the uterus is scraped with an instrument called a curette (curettage)

deficiency disease—illness caused by the absence or shortage of substances necessary to the body

degeneration—decay

diabetes—deficiency disease due to lack of insulin

diuretic—a pill for losing water

dosage—the actual amount of a drug to be given or taken

Down's syndrome—inherited chromosomal disease

drug—a medication, but not necessarily an addictive substance

dysfunction—abnormal function

dysmenorrhea—pain or cramps with menstrual period

dyspareunia—the development of pain related to sexual intercourse

edema—accumulation of fluid in the body with swelling

embryo—the early structure resulting from fertilization of sperm and egg

endocrine gland—specialized body gland that produces hormones

endocrinologist—physician specializing in hormone disorders

endometrial biopsy—sampling of uterine lining

endometriosis—disease with endometrium in body sites outside of uterus

endometrium—the lining of the uterus

enterocele—a hernia-like structure behind the uterus

environment—conditions, objects, and circumstances that surround one

ERT—estrogen replacement therapy; the popular term used for long-term estrogen treatment

estrogen—the female sex hormone produced by the ovaries

fallacy—false idea

fallopian tube—the tube from the uterus that opens near the ovary and acts as a duct for the sperm and egg

fertile—to be able to have a baby

fertilization—the joining of the egg and sperm

fetus—the baby growing inside the uterus before birth

fibroid (fibromyoma)—a fiber and muscle benign swelling of the uterus; may be multiple

flashes, hot—see hot flushes

fluid retention—see edema

follicle—sac with an egg and fluid in the ovary

fracture—the breaking of a bone

FSH—follicle stimulating hormone; a hormone secreted by the pituitary gland that stimulates the follicle in the ovary to grow

genital atrophy—the shriveling or wasting away of the female organ

genitals—the female or male sex organs

gland—body structure that secretes fluid or chemicals

gonad—sex organ containing sperm or eggs; testicle in the male and ovary in the female

gonadotropin—a hormone produced by the pituitary that can stimulate the gonad

graafian follicle—see follicle

GRH—gonadotrophin releasing hormone, the hormone made by the hypothalamus that stimulates the pituitary gland to produce gonadotropin

gynecologist—physician treating diseases of women

hormone—chemical messenger produced by the endocrine gland

hot flushes—feeling heat that spreads over arms, chest, and face

hypertension—high blood pressure

HRT—hormone replacement therapy, similar to ERT but suggests estrogen plus progestin treatment

hypothalamus—the coordinating center of the brain that lies above the pituitary gland

hysterectomy—removal of the uterus at surgery

idiosyncratic—peculiar individual reaction or characteristic

implant—hard pellet of hormone placed in the body fat under the skin, usually of estrogen, and inserted afresh every couple of months

insomnia—inability to get to sleep

intestinal malabsorption syndrome—bowel inability to absorb nutrients properly

jaundice—yellow color of the skin and eyes, usually caused by liver disease

labia major—the outer lips of the entrance to the vagina

labia minor—the inner lips of the entrance to the vagina

lactose—a form of sugar frequent in dairy products

laparoscope—a long, thin telescope for viewing inside the abdominal cavity

laparotomy—opening of the abdominal cavity surgically to explore the interior

LH—luteinizing hormone, the pituitary hormone that stimulates release of the egg from the graafian follicle and formation of the corpus luteum

libido—sexual desire and drive

lipoprotein—a complex structure of protein and fat

menarche—the first menstrual period

menopause—the final menstrual period

menstrual flow—the period, or monthly flow, of blood from the vagina

menstrual irregularity—vaginal bleeding at abnormal or irregular times

menstrual period—the monthly flow of vaginal bleeding indicating no pregnancy has occurred

menstruation—the monthly period

mortality rate—the number of deaths occurring per certain total population

natural estrogens—estrogens similar to ones made normally by the body

nausea—desire to vomit

obese—extremely fat

occlusion—blockage obstruction

oophorectomy—the removal of one or both ovaries at surgery

orgasm—the sexual climax

osteogenesis imperfecta—an inherited disease of poorly formed brittle bones

osteoporosis—thinning of bone

ovariectomy—see oophorectomy

ovary—the female organ containing eggs and making sex hormones

ovulation—escape of the egg from the graafian follicle of the ovary

PAP smear—scraping from the cervix to detect early cancerous changes

pathology—science of the study of disease in organs

pelvis—bony basin around the lower abdominal organs

perimenopause—the time around menopause; see climacteric

period—see menstruation

pessaries—vaginal medication pellets; plastic rings for supporting prolapsed uterus

pharmaceutical company—company that makes medications

pharmacology—science of the study of drugs

physiology—science of the study of functions of the body

pituitary gland—an endocrine gland located in the skull

postmenopausal—after the menopause

postmenopausal syndrome—see climacteric syndrome

premenstrual syndrome—pattern of symptoms related to menstrual cycle

primordial follicle—the early follicle in the ovary made up of the egg surrounded by cells

progesterone—one of the ovarian female hormones controlling the action of estrogen

progestin—synthetic drugs with structure and effect like progesterone

progestogen—see progestin

prolactin—hormone affecting breast produced in pituitary gland

prolapse—sagging or dropping of uterus, bladder, and vagina due to loss of pelvic support

psychogenic—problem caused by a mental rather than a physical disturbance

psychology—science of the study of behavior

puberty—transition from childhood to the reproductive age

pubic hair—the hair on the external genitals

ratio—numerical comparison between one thing and another, for example, risk to benefit

regime—plan for a course of treatment

renal failure—kidney failure

reproductive organs—ovaries, fallopian tubes, uterus, and vagina

secrete—production and release of a substance from a gland

sexual intercourse—the act of making love

side effect—an undesirable reaction produced by a drug

social—relates to the structure and way of thinking of a community

somatic—relating to the body

spotting—irregular, slight vaginal bleeding between periods

stress incontinence—inability to hold urine properly during coughing, sneezing, laughing, or exercise

subcutaneous—under the skin

surgical menopause—menopause following surgical removal of the ovaries

symptom—the feeling that alerts the body to something wrong

syndrome—a set of symptoms put together as a group

synthetic estrogens—estrogens made artificially in a laboratory

testes—the testicle or gland in the male that produces sperm

testosterone—the male hormone made by the testes

therapy—treatment

thromboembolism—breaking off of a blood clot in one part of the body and its traveling to another part via the bloodstream

tranquilizers—medications to reduce anxiety

transdermal—through the skin

urethra—the tube from the bladder through which urine escapes

uterine prolapse—see prolapse

uterus—the womb

vagina—muscular tube for sex; also the birth canal

vaginal smear—vaginal wall scraping for laboratory testing

varicose veins—dilated veins, especially of legs

vein—blood vessels carrying blood from the body to the heart

vulva—the outside of the female genitalia

womb—the uterus

Index

215

Gallstones, hormone replacement
therapy and, 91–92
Gingivectomy, 163
Glands, how they work, 23, 25
Glandular therapy, 65
Gonadotropin releasing hormone
(GRH), role of, 25
Graying of America, statistics on,
10–11
Greeks, rejuvenation and the,
65
Groote Schuur Hospital, 6

Hair
care, 164–65
removing body, 166
Harris Survey, 21
Harvard Nurses Health Study,
145
Head lift, 129
*Health Consequences of Involuntary
Smoking,* 44
Heart disease
blood pressure and, 44–45
cholesterol levels and, 42–44
cigarette smoking and, 44
heredity factors and, 40
hormone deprivation and
effects on, 39, 41
hormone replacement therapy
and, 95
obesity and, 42
prevention of, 13, 45, 81
progestin and, 69
risk factors of, 40–45
statistics on, 38–39
Height and weight tables, 193–94
Heparin, 37
High blood pressure, prevention
of, 13
High-density lipoproteins
(HDLs), 42–44
Histochemical staining, 45

Hormonal cytology, 75
Hormonal imbalances,
premenstrual syndrome and,
54, 56
Hormone replacement therapy
(HRT), 15
amount of dosages taken, 75
benefits of, 84–85, 92–97
costs, 88
creams, 71–72
differences between
progesterone and progestin,
69
frequency of, 203
future of, 77
heart disease and, 81
historical background of, 65–66
implants, 70–71
injections, 70
minimax concept and, 84
patches, 72
pills, 70
purpose of, 66
reasons for taking, 66–67
risks of, 85, 88–92
side effects of, 86–88
treatment regimens for, 72–74
types of, 68–69
vaginal creams, 71
what to expect during, 76–77
who should not have, 67–68
for women without a uterus,
75
Hormones
androgens, 182
androstenedione, 45
estrone, 45
follicle stimulating, 25
gonadotropin releasing, 25
luteinizing, 25
for premenstrual syndrome, 56
role of, 23
testosterone, 68, 154, 155